MEDITATIONS

FROM

THE MAT

MEDITATIONS FROM THE MAT

Daily Reflections on the Path of Yoga

BY ROLF GATES

AND KATRINA KENISON

ANCHOR BOOKS · A DIVISION OF RANDOM HOUSE, INC. · NEW YORK

AN ANCHOR BOOKS ORIGINAL, DECEMBER 2002

Copyright © 2002 by Rolf Gates and Katrina Kenison

Photographs by Jonathon Hexner

Anchor Books and colophon are registered trademarks of Random House, Inc.

Grateful acknowledgment is made to Harmony Books, a division of Random House, Inc. for permission to reprint an excerpt from Bhagavad Gita, translated by Stephen Mitchell. Copyright © 2000 by Stephen Mitchell. Reprinted by permission of Harmony Books, a division of Random House, Inc.

Library of Congress Cataloging-in-Publication Data
Gates, Rolf.
Meditations from the mat : daily reflections on the path of yoga / by Rolf Gates ;
edited by Katrina Kenison.
p. cm.
Includes bibliographical references.
ISBN 0-385-72154-4 (pbk.)
1. Yoga, Haòha. 2. Meditations. I. Kenison, Katrina. II. Title.
RA781.7 G376 2000
613.7'046—dc21   2002025575

Book design by Jessica Shatan

www.anchorbooks.com

Printed in the United States of America
15 17 19 20 18 16 14

TO MARIAM

By your stumbling, the world is perfected.

Sri Aurobindo

The Eight-Limb Path of Yoga

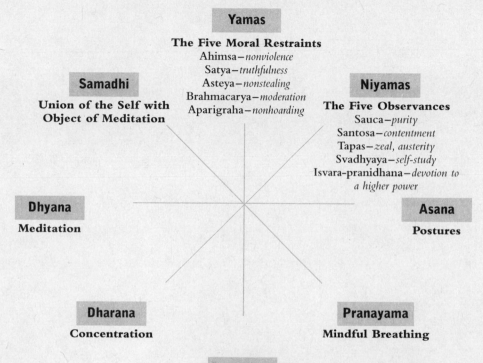

Yamas

The Five Moral Restraints
Ahimsa—*nonviolence*
Satya—*truthfulness*
Asteya—*nonstealing*
Brahmacarya—*moderation*
Aparigraha—*nonhoarding*

Samadhi

**Union of the Self with
Object of Meditation**

Niyamas

The Five Observances
Sauca—*purity*
Santosa—*contentment*
Tapas—*zeal, austerity*
Svadhyaya—*self-study*
Isvara-pranidhana—*devotion to
a higher power*

Dhyana

Meditation

Asana

Postures

Dharana

Concentration

Pranayama

Mindful Breathing

Pratyahara

Turning Inward

**The Two Aspects of
Spiritual Practice**

Abhyasa – *practice*
Vairagya – *renunciation*

The Four Aims of Life

Dharma – *observation of spiritual
discipline*
Artha – *creation of a balanced life*
Kama – *enjoyment of the fruits of
one's labors*
Moksa – *liberation*

The Five Afflictions

Avidya – *spiritual ignorance*
Asmita – *pride*
Raga – *desire*
Dvesa – *aversion*
Abhinivesa – *fear of death*

ACKNOWLEDGMENTS

I would like to begin by thanking God for the life I have been given, and my family for the love they have given me over the years. Thank you Katrina Kenison, for believing in me and in this book; Mary Evans, my agent, for impeccable advice; John Hexner, for your friendship and artistic vision; and Jenny Minton at Vintage Books, for your unwavering support. Pam Gaither, if it takes a village to raise a child, it takes great friends to write a book.

Thanks also to Baron Baptiste. Baron, our work together, our lives together, and our shared vision has been the backdrop of this book. I will be forever in your debt because you have chosen to be yourself so fully. I would also like to thank some of the other great teachers I have met along the way: Beryl Bender Birch, whose kind warrior spirit has lit my way for many years; Stephen Cope, whose passion for this work never fails to reassure me that I am on the right path; Patricia Townsend, for taking me and Mariam in when we were still wet behind the ears, and for your tremendous example; David Kennedy, whose vision of the poetry of the human experience helped to shape this book; Krishna Das, for reminding me of the Love beneath all loves; the U.S. Army Officer Corps, whose vast institutional wisdom has guided and fathered me for over half of my life; and Bill W., for everything.

My gratitude also goes to the teachers and staff at the Baptiste Power Yoga Institute: Caroline Baumal, Kate Churchill, Jeanne Coffey, Dave Emerson, Hugh Folkerth, Natalie Graber, Elizabeth Huntsman, Toby Levine, Coeli Marsh, Molly McCullough, Molly Powers, Gregor Singleton, Alyssa Sullivan, Rachel Werkman, and the Pennsylvania contingency: J. Alycia Meldon, Rhea Slichter, and Bill Raup. Words cannot express my appreciation for being numbered among you. You are my friends, my community, my support, and my inspiration.

Many thanks to Clyde Bergstresser, Daniel Boyne, Neena Buck, Gil Clothey, Vicki Evarts, Sudhir Jonathan Foust, Leigh Hare, Amy Lewis, Martha Mueller, Jene' Rossi, Laura Scileppi, Roman Szpond, Eleanor Williams, and the others who have already been mentioned, who took the time to share their stories here and enrich our lives. To all of the students I have met along the way, thank you for showing up. Finally, thanks to my wife Mariam for all the hours you have spent with me helping to bring this book into the world. Without your support it would not have been written.

CONTENTS

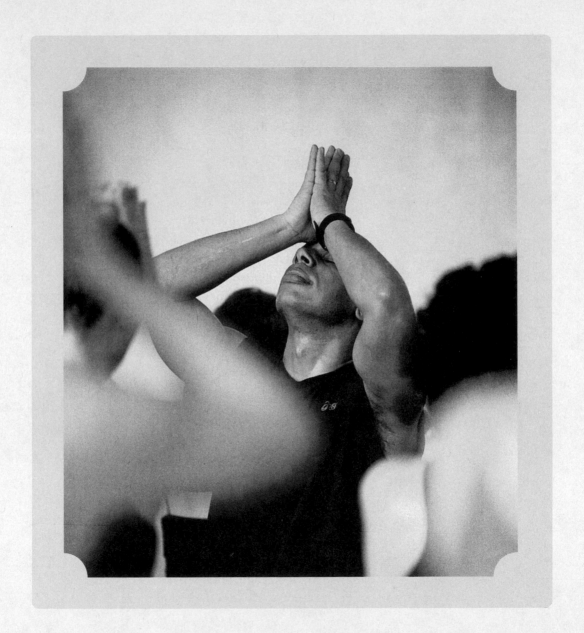

INTRODUCTION

Future generations, riding on the highways that we built,
I hope they have a better understanding.

John Cougar Mellencamp

All of us carry a desire for a better way, a hope that we will somehow leave the world a better place than we found it. Whether we practice yoga or meditation, vote Democratic or Republican, write popular music or computer code, we cherish the notion that things can improve and that our own good life contributes in some way to the good lives of those who will come after us. Moreover, we live in the presence of men and women who *have* made the world a better place and who seem to have achieved some measure of inner peace in the process. Human history is replete with good lives lived despite, or possibly because of, overwhelming adversity.

Nevertheless, for the vast majority of us the path is not always clear. John Cougar Mellencamp writes about his *hope* for the future, not his certainty that the next generation will do a better job of living than we have. How easy it is to move through our days as if we were in some sort of dress rehearsal for real life—despite the nagging suspicion that this is *it,* that real life is right here, right now. How, then, shall we make it count? How do we find our way? Such uncertainty is part of the human condition and always has been. In response to this age-old questioning, this yearning for clarity and direction, we humans have, over the centuries, created a vast multitude of paths and called them by many names—religions, philosophies, political ideologies. Yoga is one path out of the spiritual wilderness, a highway that was built by those who came before us and that has been trodden by millions over thousands of years. This book is for anyone who chooses to join those millions and explore yoga as a road home to a better understanding.

I came to yoga in an ordinary way: my girlfriend (now my wife) dragged me to a weekend retreat. I had attended a few classes with her before, but yoga really took hold for me at a 6 A.M. class at the Kripalu Center in western Massachusetts. I remember very little of the class itself, except that I was asked to do something odd with my nose, which I later learned was *pranayama,* or breath control. What stood out for me at the time was the way I felt as I walked down the hall to breakfast afterward. It was without a doubt the best walk to breakfast I had ever experienced. I had a joy in my body that decades of sports and devotion to exercise had never been able to provide. The seed had been planted. In the following years I practiced yoga daily, simply because it made me feel better. I was working with young people who were in a good deal of pain, and I found that yoga made it possible for me to show up, physically and emotionally, day after day. Yoga was profoundly effective self-care.

Eventually I enrolled in a teacher training program in order to deepen my own practice. I wanted to be able to take my yoga with me wherever I went. A year later, out of the blue, I was offered a job teaching yoga. An inner voice seemed to be telling me that it was important that I teach yoga. This voice had spoken to me only once before, assuring me that everything was going to be OK, at a time in my life when absolutely nothing was. The voice had proved right the first time, and so I listened to it again. Despite the fact that I was already busy with graduate school and a job, I taught my butt off. I taught in gyms, karate studios, health clubs, boardrooms, and living rooms. Something told me I needed to teach as much as possible. There were some fine affirming moments, too—connections with students, the quiet during *shavasana,* the deep rest at the end of class, the sense of doing something ancient and good. But there was also something missing.

About the time I was running out of steam, an impassioned teacher named Baron Baptiste came to Cambridge and opened a studio. He captured my imagination immediately. His first words to me, after I had taken one of his classes, were a question: "Are you a teacher?" I said I was, but the words didn't ring true. I taught classes but I was not a teacher. I went to work for Baron, and I became a teacher.

The word "educator" comes from the Latin verb *educere,* which means to lead forth or draw out. The Latin term was used by midwives, with the meaning "to be present at the birth of." From Baron I learned that teaching yoga is first and foremost about drawing forth that which is already in a student. Alignment, breath, a sequence of postures—these are simply the tools with which the teacher grabs the student's attention. If education is really the art of helping to develop each individual's innate capacities, then teaching yoga becomes much more than a rote litany of poses and explanations. I became a teacher in the true sense when I recognized my teaching as a divine opportunity to be present at the birth of an individual's authentic self. The real payoff of a yoga practice, I came to see, is not a perfect handstand or a deeper forward bend—it is the newly born self that each day steps off the yoga mat and back into life.

Soon after, I left the graduate social work program I was in and became a full-time yoga teacher. I had found my path of service. *A Course in Miracles* says, "To teach is to demonstrate." As far as I can tell, the only thing worth demonstrating is love. Now I spend my days demonstrating love to the extraordinary individuals who come to my studio. It has been a profound experience and an ongoing education.

If you are like most of the students I know, you probably arrived at your first yoga class without any background in yoga philosophy and without any interest in it, either. As the months passed, however, you began to experience the benefits of a regular yoga practice. You started to internalize the bits and pieces of yoga philosophy you were hearing in class, you began to feel better, life seemed more manageable, you felt happier. Aches and pains you may have suffered for decades mysteriously evaporated. Limiting beliefs you'd held about your physical shape and lack of ability began to be challenged and gradually went the way of your disappearing back pain and stiff hips.

Over time, a hunger develops. Yoga class gives us a taste of a new way to be in the world, a new way of moving, a new way of responding to daily events and challenges. Eventually we want to bring more of what yoga has to offer into our daily lives. I do not have enough hours in the week to teach all the private classes and extra sessions students ask of me. By and large, these are people just like you, people who are simply trying to get a bit more yoga into their lives. The physical part is already happening in class; what they are asking for now is the spiritual part. They would like to spend some one-on-one time with a teacher, to have a chance to ask their questions, and to be joined, even if only for an hour or two, on their new journey. And so would we all.

This book is a response to that need for companionship. Yoga is essentially a journey inward. Whether we squeeze into a class of seventy, practice alone in front of a video, or pair up with a partner at the beach, we all experience solitary periods in our practice. We are often far from the support of our teachers when we practice yoga, and further still from their guidance as we seek to truly live our yoga from one moment to the next.

As an orienteer in the military I learned to habitually confirm my position, every hundred yards or so, whether I thought I needed to or not. The first reading was always the most important, however, because all subsequent calculations followed from it. If you're going to navigate through the wilderness, you've got to know your start point. It is my hope that this book will be your daily start point. As you read each day's reflection, I invite you to take that moment to be still, to get your bearings, to plan your day's journey.

The pieces that follow are a natural outgrowth of the work that goes on in any yoga studio. Awakening our limbs, breathing deeply into our muscles, opening our hearts, we are stirred to look more deeply into our souls. What I bring to these pages is my own practice, my own journey, and my own commitment to teach you by drawing forth that which is already within you. I will not have answers for all your questions, nor will I tell you how to stand in triangle pose or point your toes in shoulder stand. Instead we will travel side by side through the days of the year, observing the seasons of our practice and the discoveries we make both on and off the mat. Here, then, is a bit of one-on-one time with a teacher, a start point for the day as you prepare to travel this five-thousand-year-old path called yoga.

If you read the essays in order, you will see that they build on one another, and the whole will make sense to you. I invite you to read this book over the course of a year, one essay a day. Or read a couple of pages at a time, in moments when you need guidance and inspiration. Do whatever works for you, but read slowly, and take time to digest the ideas. Allow the momentum of this book to build in your life, to overflow into your practice, your work, your relationships, your experience of being alive.

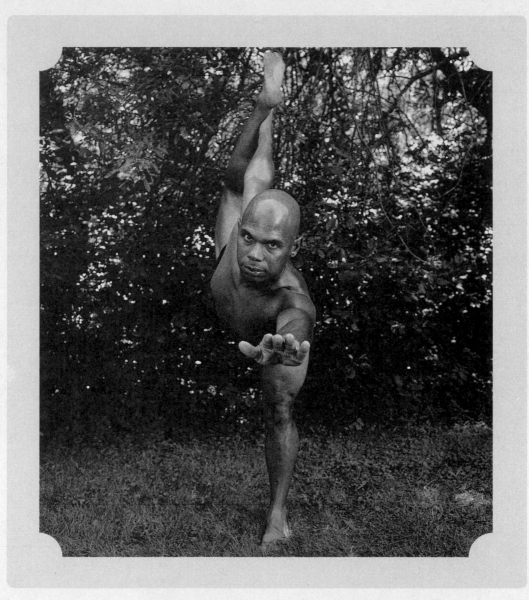

PART ONE

THE YAMAS

The Beginning

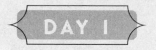

DAY 1

He that will not apply new remedies must expect new evils;
for time is the greatest innovator.

Sir Francis Bacon

As we move into the twenty-first century, yoga seems to be the West's new remedy. Yet this remedy is in fact over five thousand years old—far older than Islam, even older than Christianity. Today, in yoga studios throughout the West, Sanskrit, one of the oldest written languages, is used as contemporary classroom jargon. So we might ask, Why yoga? And why now?

I believe our hunger for yoga, and our eagerness to embrace yoga as a spiritual practice, are a testament to our growth and our desire for change. In the aftermath of the bloodbath that was the twentieth century, and in the presence of threats posed by more recent events, there is a pressing need for what Buddhist scholar Robert Thurman describes as a "cold revolution." We need a new paradigm, one that will replace our present attachment to imbalance. Yoga is the study of balance, and balance is the aim of all living creatures; it is our home.

The flow of this book follows the course of Patanjali's Yoga Sutras. Written between 500 and 200 B.C., the Sutras codified a spiritual path that was already many centuries old at the time the Sutras were actually written down. Patanjali provides 196 succinct lessons on the nature of the human condition, human potential, and how that potential can be realized. Comprehensive, systematic, and remarkably precise, the Yoga Sutras organize the essence of all spiritual practices into a basic plan for living. You will find nothing in this ancient text that contradicts the precepts of any religion. Instead you will find a step-by-step guide to right living, a guide that complements the goals of any spiritual tradition.

PART ONE

The Beginning

1

A spiritual practice is one that brings us full circle—not to a new self but, rather, back to the essence of our true selves. Yoga is the practice of celebrating what is. At the end of the hero's journey, he finds that he did not need to go anywhere, that all he sought was inside him all along. Dorothy, having traveled across time and space to the land of Oz, and having struggled desperately to find her way back to Kansas, discovers that she could have gone home at any time. In the end, she learns that her adventures have simply brought her to the point where she can believe this. It is the aim of all spiritual seeking to bring us home, home to the understanding that we already have everything we need.

We are far now from home, and weary from our travels. The sun is setting and there is no destination in sight. Yoga is a lamp lit in the window of our home, dimly glimpsed across the spiritual wilderness in which we wander. At a time when we could not feel further from our home, yoga reminds us that we are already there, that we need simply awaken from our dream of separation, our dream of imperfection. Allow this book to awaken you, to be a light that shines in the darkness, guiding you through your days, pointing you home.

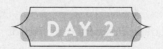

Burning zeal in practice, self-study and study of scriptures, and surrender to God are the acts of yoga.

B. K. S. Iyengar

The Yoga Sutras outline a plan for living that flows from action to knowledge to liberation. This plan, or path, has eight limbs, which work more like spokes on a wheel than like steps on a ladder. The first four limbs are the limbs of *tapas,* or spirituality in action. Included here are the *yamas* and the *niyamas,* or the five moral restraints and five observances of yoga. The *yamas* and *niyamas* are akin to the Ten Commandments and are the true foundation of the yoga student's life.

The next two limbs of *tapas* are asana and *pranayama,* the postures and yogic breathing. The *yamas* and *niyamas,* asana, and *pranayama* all combine to form our path of action as we deepen our practice. They are actions taken or not taken with our bodies.

The *yamas* and *niyamas* bring us into right relationship with ourselves, others, and the spirit of the universe. The asana refine our bodies, deepen our awareness of the senses, and enhance our powers of concentration. In *pranayama* we develop control over the flow of our breath, thereby entering into a dance with our life energy. These four practices refresh the body, refine the mind, and bring peace to the heart, allowing us to meet the pressures of life with equanimity.

The next two limbs of the eight-limb path are called *svadhyaya,* or self-study. They are *pratyahara* and *dharana. Pratyahara* literally means turning inward—the mind withdraws from the senses of perception. In the stillness of *pratyahara, dharana*—or concentration—can be developed. The light of our awareness can begin to shine on our soul. The deepest form of connectedness is now possible.

Dhyana and *samadhi* form the final spokes of the wheel and comprise the limbs of *isvara,* the final frontier—the surrender of the individual self to the universal self. *Dhyana* is meditation, and *samadhi* is union with the object of meditation—the state in which meditation is no longer necessary, in which we reexperience our primal oneness, we come home.

The eight limbs are a map, but in yoga as in life, the journey is more important than the destination. In Alcoholics Anonymous they say that "we must be willing to grow along spiritual lines." And that is really all that is necessary as we undertake a yoga practice. We must simply remain open to our own spiritual potential and be willing to take action on our own behalf.

As the days go by, we will examine each aspect of the eight-limb path in turn. Together we will experience the great adventure, the only adventure, the journey from darkness into light.

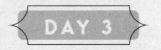

Everything all the time . . .

The Eagles

At first glance, the eight-limb path appears to lend itself to a linear approach. It would seem to make sense: you do the first limb, then you proceed to the second, and so on. In fact, we take up all the limbs together. As the line in the Eagles song goes, we do everything all the time. It's not possible to practice the first two limbs, the *yamas* and the *niyamas,* without the support of the practices outlined by the other limbs. As we practice asana and *pranayama,* the postures and breath work that comprise the third and fourth limbs, we refine our relationship to our body, creating the necessary circumstances for *brahmacarya,* or moderation, the fourth *yama.* To practice living in the truth, or *satya,* the second *yama,* we must have a mind that has let go of the habit of distraction and developed the habit of concentration. Concentration is deliberately cultivated in *dharana,* the sixth limb. We must actually do everything all the time.

Our yoga practice makes this possible. Each time we come to the mat, we have an opportunity to work the entire path, moment by moment. As we move through the postures we are constantly enacting each aspect of the path. Our bodies, our breath, our minds, and our choices are being refined in the laboratory that is our yoga mat. As this symphony becomes established on our mats, it becomes established in our lives as well. Driving to work, mailing a letter, meeting a friend for lunch all become part of the uninterrupted flow of our yoga practice. We are doing our yoga all the time.

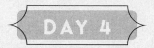

We are the ones we've been waiting for.

Hopi elder

Now that you have a sense of how the book will flow, go with it. The Yoga Sutras will set the course as, in our travels, we explore each tributary of the eight-limb path. The daily readings that follow are an invitation to get into the canoe of your practice and flow down the river of yoga. You may go deep, into uncharted waters; you will surely encounter challenges and delights along the way. But first you must get into that canoe and let go. In class I say, Let your practice be a refuge from the need to control. And I suggest the same to you: get out of the driver's seat for a while and enjoy the scenery. Let the river of yoga take you where it will. If you hit whitewater, stay in the canoe and keep paddling. When you enter calm pools, do the same.

At a Native American gathering in Arizona for the 1999 summer solstice, a Hopi elder said: "There is a river flowing now, very fast. It is so great and swift that there are those who will be afraid. They will try to hold on to the shore. They will feel they are being torn apart and suffer greatly. Know that the river has its destination. The elders say we must push off into the middle of the river, keep our eyes open and our heads above the water. See who is in there with you and celebrate. At this time in history we are to take nothing personally, least of all ourselves, for the moment we do that, our spiritual growth comes to a halt. The time of the lone wolf is over. Gather yourselves; banish the word 'struggle' from your attitude and vocabulary. All that we do now must be done in a sacred way and in celebration. We are the ones we've been waiting for."

Now, go to your mat and push off from the shore.

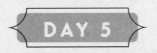

When transgressions hinder, the weight of the imagination should be thrown on the other side.

Yoga Sutras

In a reflection of the pragmatism that is at the core of all yoga teachings, Patanjali takes a moment, before he begins to outline the necessary restraints of yoga, to tell us what to do if we get into trouble along the way. Whenever we find ourselves ensnared in negative behavior, he suggests, we should increase the amount of time, thought, and energy we direct toward positive behavior. This simple, elegant notion is articulated by Marianne Williamson in her spiritual guidebook *A Return to Love*. "If you want to end darkness," she writes, "you cannot beat it with a baseball bat, you have to turn on a light." We do not need to enter a showdown with our self-destructive behavior, nor can we deny its existence. We must simply come to know it, and move on. We learn to focus wholeheartedly on positive behavior.

Reading Deepak Chopra's *The Seven Spiritual Laws of Success,* I came to understand that my own "What's in it for me?" attitude—however subtle or well disguised—was blocking me professionally. Chopra suggests that one of the simplest ways to access grace in any situation is to ask, "How can I be helpful?" Once I saw that my typical M.O. is to ask, "What's in it for me?"

I did not enter into a protracted struggle to obliterate the question from my psyche. Instead, I simply embarked on the magnificent journey that begins with the question "How can I be helpful?" As soon as I began to direct my energy and attention to a new question, the old one fell away. The Yoga Sutras suggest that we deliberately turn away from the choice for death and embrace the choice for life.

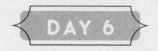

DAY 6

If you do what you did, you get what you got.

Anonymous

The Yoga Sutras lay out two aspects of spiritual practice: *abhyasa,* practice, and *vairagya,* nonattachment or renunciation. Over two thousand years later, the notions of practice and renunciation are reflected in the twelve-step adage "If you do what you did, you get what you got." Renunciation on its own has no staying power. You can renounce bananas all you like, but if you continue to live in your banana home on your banana street, if you keep your job at the banana warehouse and hang out with your banana-gobbling friends, you'll be eating bananas before you know it. Practice is doing the work. It is following up your intention with action.

Many of us attend a few yoga classes and find that we like the glimpse of another way of life that yoga offers. We are delighted by the way we feel after class and we are pleasantly surprised as certain behaviors start to fall away. Perhaps we no longer need coffee in the morning; or staying out late at night becomes less attractive; or we find ourselves calmer and more compassionate. Suddenly we're convinced that we've hit upon a painless way to solve all our problems. Sadly, this is not the case. Practice is not a substitute for the difficult work of renunciation. The postures and breath work that you do in a typical yoga class *will* change your life. These practices—asana and *pranayama*—suffuse us with the energy we need to take on the hard choices and to endure the inevitable highs and lows. What yoga practice will not do, however, is take the place of the hard lessons each of us has to learn in order to mature spiritually. Renunciation is the acid test; it is walking the walk.

A number of my students come to yoga with issues concerning food and body image. Some binge, some starve, some purge; some do all of the above; some just obsess to the point that it blocks their personal growth. In each case there needs to be an ending and a new beginning. The old behavior must be faced and renounced. Yoga practice is not a substitute for that all-important process, but it does support us as we make a commitment to change. Once we take the first step of renunciation, our practice nourishes and sustains us as we are reborn. Practice without renunciation is avoidance. Renunciation without practice is not long-lived. Together, practice and renunciation make all our dreams possible.

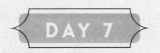

DAY 7

Every blade of grass has its angel that bends over it and whispers, "Grow, grow."

The Talmud

Many of us have spent years trying to ameliorate the world's suffering without first confronting our own. The belief that it is possible to heal the world without healing ourselves first is what the Yoga Sutras call a lack of true knowledge. The truth is, when we are happy we spread happiness, and when we are in pain we spread suffering. If our aim is to alleviate the world's suffering, we must begin with our own minds and bodies. We must do yoga. Each action taken in compliance with the eight-limb path brings with it an increase in our own peace and happiness—and our happiness is welcomed by the universe. We do not need to fear the steps we are about to take. In fact, we will experience each right action, no matter how small or insignificant, as a pleasure and a relief. With each step we take toward the light, the universe rejoices. When we let go of our suffering, we participate in the salvation of all living beings.

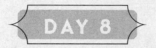

DAY 8

Vairagya is the elimination of whatever hinders progress and refinement.

B. K. S. Iyengar

In a culture of more, it is hard to sell the concept of less. Thoreau wrote, "A man is rich in proportion to the number of things which he can afford to let alone." He knew intuitively that through nonaction we can gain the power we seek. Fortunately, yoga is a reality-based philosophy. Everywhere we turn, we see examples of yoga in action. The yogic requirement that we move through life shedding self-defeating behaviors does not need to be explained or defended. If you're reading this book, chances are you've already been practicing *vairagya,* or letting go, for some time, whether consciously or not. This simple concept has merited so much elaboration in yogic texts over the years because we seem to have been born with a propensity for vacillation. Given a choice, we tend to hold on.

It is human nature to obfuscate, rationalize, temporize, overanalyze, generalize, minimize. When we make a commitment to our practice, though, the obstacles to our progress suddenly come into clear focus. Then we are called upon to practice *vairagya*. The *Tao Te Ching* tells us, "In the pursuit of knowledge, every day something is added. In the practice of the Tao, every day something is dropped." So it is as we begin to live our yoga—there is a sense of liberation and lightness as we begin to renounce the very things that have held us back.

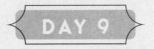

DAY 9

We are beaten and blown by the wind, blown by the wind,
oh when I go there, I go there with you, it's all I can do.

U2

About six months after I began my spiritual practice in earnest, my older sister committed suicide. She was thirty-one years old, and I loved her more than anyone on earth. I had just come home from the service and I was living with her and her new husband. She was young, healthy, and successful, and I worshiped her. After her death, her husband and I grew closer. We had been playing racquetball together and we continued to do so, supporting each other as best we could. Then, within weeks of my sister's death, Peter showed me a lump on his chest one night before we began to play. As it turned out, he had cancer. When he gave me the news, we just looked at each other. There was nothing to say. Two months before, we had been talented young men with the world at our feet. Now, it seemed, we were living our own worst nightmares.

A few weeks later, as we were on our way to the gym, I came to understand the true meaning of the word *abhyasa*, or practice. *Abhyasa* refers not only to yogic practice but also to the attitude with which a practice is approached. *Abhyasa* is unconditional. It is the dedicated, unswerving application of what you believe in. I was driving along behind Peter, in a car I had bought in Europe a few years before—a vestige of another life. A song by U2 came on my radio. Watching Peter drive, up ahead of me, I heard the words "We are beaten and blown by the wind, blown by the wind, oh and when I go there, I go there with you, it's all I can do."

Both of us, I realized, had surrendered completely to the God of our understanding. Despite the terrific beating we were experiencing at the hands of fate, each of us was still living out his faith. Even in the presence of extraordinary pain, we were taking right action, we were attending to our practice, each in his own way. As I listened to the lyrics of this song, the depth of my commitment to my own spiritual path became clear to me. My sister's death was certainly not in any bargain I had made concerning my spiritual life. Any hopes that spirituality would be a primrose path had been dashed. What I understood in that moment was that at some deep level, both my brother-in-law and I had made a decision—we had committed unconditionally to our practice. This commitment was not about results, and it would hold up under the gravest challenges. I don't know exactly when I made that decision, or if the decision actually made me. I do believe *abhyasa* is not something we earn or achieve through force of will; rather, it is an innate human capacity that we awaken through practice, through our own willingness. It is an energy that builds in our lives as we use it. And it will be there for us in hard times if we cultivate it in good times.

PART ONE

The Beginning

13

DAY 10

I had seen birth and death,
But had thought they were different; this Birth was
Hard and bitter agony for us, like Death, our death.
We returned to our places, these Kingdoms,
But no longer at ease here, in the old dispensation . . .

T. S. Eliot

In this beautiful passage from "Journey of the Magi," one of the three wise men recalls his experience of the birth of Christ. His revelation captures a powerful aspect of *vairagya,* or renunciation. Before we are truly ready to renounce something, renunciation seems like a pointless sacrifice. "Sure," we tell ourselves, "I'd love to take a run every morning, but I really prefer to sleep in."

But then there is a shift in perception. The furniture of our life gets moved, and we are forced to pay attention. In the experience of the magi, a birth signals the death of their old way of life. More often than not, however, this shift in our perceptions is associated with some kind of loss—a literal death, or the death of some aspect of our false self. We may lose a coveted opportunity; or a door that we thought would always be open unexpectedly slams shut. Suddenly we are seeing the world with new eyes. In the wake of this death, we are born to a new understanding. We are no longer at ease with the old dispensations. We look at our friends, our habits, our choices, and see them all in the new light, as all our old assumptions fall away.

The soil of our life is ready for *vairagya.* Now that I've told you that renunciation is an aspect of the yoga path, you may be thinking that I keep a hair shirt in the back of my closet and that I'm about to ask you to wear one, too. But it is important to remember that the nature of all lasting change is less radical. Long before we actually die to an old behavior, the way has been paved for a new one. By the time we actually arrive at the decision to let go of something, we shall "be glad of another death." When we are ready to let go, we will do so with relief. We will experience renunciation not as a death but as a birth.

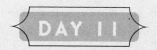

DAY 11

The master sticks to her tools.

Lao-Tzu

Lao-Tzu captured the essence of *abhyasa,* or practice. We get the job, we don't get the job; we get married, we don't get married; our family is well, our family is troubled; our friends flourish, our friends founder; our demons are melting away, our demons are at the door; we wake up with a love for life, we wake up filled with free-floating anxiety; we feel worthy of the love in our life, we feel unworthy of the love in our life. . . . Through it all, though, we come back to the mat, we return to the meditation cushion, we do the next right thing.

Oftentimes I feel unworthy of my practice. I remember the lofty, virtuous times of my practice, and I compare those times to my present lame condition. Pretty soon, I feel as though I don't even deserve to practice. Other days, I am on top of the world; I get it, I truly *get* it—the world needs me, and meeting my destiny is even more important than my practice. And then there are times when I am on the middle road; I am right sized and my practice is right sized. But I cannot wait around for those middle-road times. If I am not practicing right along, through all the highs and lows, I will never return to the middle road.

My very first practice was abstinence from alcohol through the use of the twelve steps. When I was about two years into that practice, a woman asked me what I wanted in life. I told her that in twenty-five years I wanted to be twenty-seven years sober. She told me that if I continued to feel that way, it would probably come to pass. *Abhyasa,* or practice, is really about making something a priority. As we enact that priority, an energy builds in our life to support it.

When I first got sober I was astounded to hear about homeless people who drank every day for years. I just did not understand how they could afford it! What I failed to realize is the power of making something a priority. If drinking is your priority, you will find a way to do it whether you have a roof over your head or not.

By choosing to practice yoga, we are saying that our spiritual growth is important to us. We are making it a priority. Our practice is a shelter we build for our spiritual selves. It is the work that we do to safeguard and support the possibility of spiritual growth. The winds of life constantly wear away at this shelter, but if we stick to our tools, the shelter will hold.

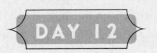

DAY 12

Do everything with a mind that has let go.

John Chan

I rarely teach a class that doesn't include at least one student who is brand-new to yoga. Working with beginners affords me an excellent opportunity to observe just what it is we bring to our mats. Despite wide age, gender, socioeconomic, cultural, and physical differences, we all carry some of the same baggage. Whether you are a dancer, a housewife, a grad student, a retired police officer, or an aerobics dropout, you will no doubt confront the same roadblocks to learning that I see students encounter every day: pride and fear.

If you are new to yoga, chances are you are wrestling not only with the postures but also with the judgments you pronounce on your efforts. But if you can make a commitment to be a little easier on yourself, I am certain you will enjoy your practice more. If not, you may soon find yourself making all sorts of excuses to avoid practicing altogether—it will become just too painful.

When we opt out of experiences that challenge us, it's usually because our pride is in the way. And "pride" is really another word for fear—the fear of not being enough. Marlon Brando delivers this truth magnificently in *Apocalypse Now* when, sweating in a nadir of spiritual bankruptcy, he tells his executioner, "It is our judgment that defeats us." We become our own executioners when we sit in judgment of our efforts. Only when we act without judgment can we truly flourish in our lives. Yoga means becoming one. As long as we stand apart in judgment, we sabotage the opportunity for connection and integration that is yoga. So I encourage you: get into that canoe and ride with the river. Commit and don't look back. Before our bodies can open, they must first let go; the clenched and guarded muscles must relax. But the mind must let go first.

PART ONE

The Beginning

17

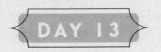

DAY 13

The first step in this process of mindful awareness is
radical self-acceptance.

Stephen Batchelor

Before we consider the necessary restraints of yoga, I would like to rein-force an important aspect of the work ahead. Buddhist teachings remind us that what we resist persists. For most of us—steeped as we are in the Judeo-Christian concepts of sin and guilt—our early efforts to examine our fear, pride, lust, ambition, avarice, perfectionism, or whatever else, are often sab-otaged by our reaction to being human. Throughout my own spiritual journey, the behavior that has caused me the most suffering is not my anger, but my anger at having become angry in the first place. Stuck in this cycle of anger begetting more anger, the best I can do is check out of a situation, depart before creating more damage, and return later, still feeling bad, to apologize. My reaction to my anger stems from the assumption that I am not supposed to have anger. If I were being spiritual, I scold myself, then I wouldn't *get* angry. I become incensed that I have allowed myself and my circumstances to get so out of control.

We do not have to succumb to the tyranny of our own self-judgment. We can observe our reactions with awareness, and let them go. Over the years I've come to realize that spiritual practice is not about locking up all the unruly aspects of myself, in the hope that they will never get free. Spir-itual practice is about turning on the light—and the light is love.

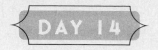

DAY 14

Don't throw the baby out with the bathwater.

Old proverb

In yoga we learn to stay with the posture, to hold the posture. Difficulty, discomfort, fear, boredom, distraction—the entire gamut of thoughts and emotions arises, and we simply observe their comings and goings. We learn to use what comes up to inform the present posture and to help us in the postures to come. There is a liability in this ethos, however, thanks to our "No pain, no gain" Puritan heritage. The hardworking, well-intentioned yoga student often believes that nothing less than a 100 percent, gonads-to-the-wall effort will do. The fallout from this misconception can be injury, but more often it is simply bitterness and blame. We may blame our teachers for teaching too hard a class, but more often we will blame ourselves for simply not being better than we are. On good days we feel the elation of living up to our expectations; the bad days are fraught with frustration and failure. Caught in this negative cycle of judgment and evaluation, we find ourselves, at best, blocked from the most nourishing aspects of yoga, and at worst, unable to sustain our practice. Defeated, we give up and move on, believing we have failed and that yoga is not for us.

There is another way. We need to learn to make rest a part of our practice, and we need to take that rest long before we feel exhausted or frustrated. Beginners can rest and regroup in child's pose, taking a few calming breaths before moving on to the next posture. If you begin to think of rest periods as an active part of your practice, you will stay in tune with what your body is telling you, and act accordingly. Intermediate students can learn to rest in the posture itself. This is an important concept. We enter a posture, the heat builds, and before long we want to get the heck out of

Dodge. That is one option—retreat. But another option is to just back off a little within the posture, rest for a breath or two, and then see if you can deepen the pose.

As a young man I would look in awe at older people around me who could sustain their effort at a job or a project over many years. I didn't realize that these men and women had learned to rest in the posture.

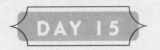

DAY 15

A state in which the aspirant is one with the object
of his meditation.

B. K. S. Iyengar, describing *samadhi*

I recently read a description of the training that Crazy Horse, the famous Sioux warrior, received as a young boy. During the day he would roam the plains with his friends, learning to hunt, ride, and take care of himself while also providing food for the less fortunate in his community. In the evening his father would question him closely on every detail of what he had seen that day: Which side of the trees had lighter bark? Which side had more regular branches? What was the meaning of the jay's call? When the swallows flew, were their mouths full, or empty? A nineteenth-century Native American living on the plains knew the medicinal properties of more than two thousand plants. The manner in which this education was achieved was simple—the young Native American was expected to pay attention to the living beings in his world, to actually see what he was looking at.

In yoga, the first step when we enter a posture is to establish our gaze. Our eyes literally rest at one point. The gaze is mindful; we are meant to actually see what we are looking at. Yoga uses the senses—sight, sound, sensation—to bring us into the present. This practice of *drishti,* or gaze point, is the same as the old Native American practice of teaching children to see what they are looking at. As a species we have a wondrous heritage of connectedness, of communion, of being present, of celebrating the fact that we are at once engulfed by and at one with the divine. Our yoga practice allows us to participate in this tradition. Our willingness to see what we are looking at allows us to perpetuate it.

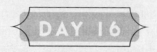

DAY 16

Half measures availed us nothing.

Alcoholics Anonymous

I once heard a story about a group of monks going down to a river at night, getting in a boat, and rowing as hard as they could. At dawn they discovered that they had made no progress. They had forgotten to untie the boat. To me, this anecdote beautifully illustrates the importance of the *yamas* and *niyamas,* the moral restraints and observances of yoga. Most Americans have their first introduction to yoga in a class. These classes are, in fact, asana classes. That is, they are yoga posture classes. The asana, or postures, are the third limb of the eight-limb path. The *yamas* and *niyamas* are the first and second limbs of the path and form the foundation of all the work that follows.

So, for those of us who did not come to yoga with a mature spiritual practice already in place, there is a missing piece, even from the very beginning. Oftentimes this sense that something is missing manifests in a desire for more: more yoga postures, harder yoga postures, more classes per week, more workshops, more teachers, more styles, more technique. There is a restlessness—out with the old routine, in with the new yoga routine; out with the old job, in with the new job on the healing path; out with the old community of friends, in with the new yoga pals. But our new awareness only serves to deepen our sense that something is not right. Our restlessness and our desire for more are actually useful indicators of our need for change. What we need is not to dig a new well, but to dig even more deeply the well we are already in.

The means for digging deeper are the *yamas* and *niyamas*. These are the tools that will support our transformation. The *yamas* and *niyamas* provide us with the energy, the balance, the necessary insight, and the motivation to work the rest of the limbs of the path. The eight-limb path is not linear; it is a dance of energies building upon themselves. But without the *yamas* and the *niyamas,* the rest of the path is empty technique. Practicing without the full engagement of our hearts and souls, we are like the monks tied to the dock.

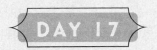

Let us not love in word or speech but in deed and in truth.

John 3:18

The first four limbs of yoga—the *yamas,* the *niyamas,* asana, and *pranayama*—are love in action. The *yamas* and the *niyamas,* specifically, are love "in deed and in truth." Tomorrow we will embark on the never-ending journey of the *yamas,* the first limb of yoga, the necessary restraints of a spiritual life. The *yamas* and *niyamas* reflect the yogic balance of *abhyasa,* or practice, and *vairagya,* nonattachment. The *yamas* are those renunciations to be embraced, and the *niyamas* are practices to be cultivated. Together they lay the foundation for effective living.

As you prepare for this journey, it is important to remember that we are simply eliminating blocks to our progress and cultivating the energy we need for our spiritual growth. This is not a test, and you will not be found lacking. The ashram where I first fell in love with yoga was led by a wonderful yogi, an accomplished man who had practiced yoga for most of his life. Unfortunately, he brought the community he had built crashing down around him, the result of not adhering to a number of the *yamas.* As I see it, this man did not fail, nor was he able to avoid the painful consequences of his actions. He did hurt many people, but he did not fail. He is alive today, he continues to practice yoga, and he continues to have the opportunity to learn from his past mistakes and to make better choices, as implied in the *yamas* and *niyamas.*

The *yamas* and *niyamas* would not be needed if we—the entire human race—did not already have the propensity to violate them. Paradoxically, the *yamas* and *niyamas* would not be possible to uphold if our true essence were not love, if love were not our aim and our home. To practice the *yamas* and *niyamas* we must find within ourselves the maturity to tolerate the duality of our nature, while allowing the possibility of victory over our darkness. Love is not a thought, it is an action. And each loving action that we take infuses us with more energy for loving action in the future.

When nonviolence in speech, thought, and action is established, one's aggressive nature is relinquished and others abandon hostility in one's presence.

Yoga Sutras

The first *yama*—*ahimsa,* or nonharming, which asks us to embrace nonviolence at the level of speech, thought, and action—is a profound and radical concept that is truly the cornerstone of yoga as a way of life. The practice of *ahimsa* could not be further from the training I received as a young man. Everything in the world in which I grew up validated competition, struggle, the annihilation of one's enemies. As a wrestler, my favorite activity was to go away to another school and vanquish some hometown favorite in front of his disheartened fans. As a young cadet, I heard an army Ranger recruiter explain that the Rangers specialized in missions that entailed a high degree of shock and violence. I said to myself, "Now that is very cool," and I signed on. I've been asked innumerable times how someone who started out as I did, willing to kill on command, ended up where I am now, devoting my life to a path of nonharming. In fact, the leap is not as great as people think it is. It is simply a matter of perception. As a man of violence, I genuinely thought I was doing the right thing—and so, for that matter, did everyone around me. As a young man I did exactly what our society tells young men to do, and I performed my service with devotion.

What changed was that I survived long enough to begin to develop my own ideas of right and wrong. As a young person I embraced the values of those around me as my own. With time and life experience, though, I began to develop my own understanding. What I've kept from my childhood and young adulthood is the concept of service. What I have discarded is the idea that there are good people and bad people, people who should be helped and people who should be killed. A friend of mine told me of a guru from Sri Lanka who was asked, "What will be the undoing of humanity?" He answered: "The separation between you and me." *Ahimsa* asks us to abandon the notion of separation.

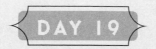

DAY 19

Well, darkness has a hunger that's insatiable, and lightness has a call that's hard to hear.

Indigo Girls

I read recently that a new war crime has been added to the list of crimes the United Nations is prosecuting. I spent some time digesting this information, willing myself to envision its victims and to imagine its perpetrators as my brothers and sisters. I tried to feel for a moment the suffering of human beings lost in the living hell that is war. My work with children and families in the relatively quiet towns and cities of the United States has given me a sense of the universality of that suffering. There is no end to it, and we minimize this truth, or believe that we are somehow disconnected from it, at our own peril.

Not long ago, a friend of mine went to a gas station to call for help with her drug problem. She couldn't use the phone in her apartment because she had already sold it for drugs. A few months later, after cleaning up her act a little, she went back to using drugs—only to experience far greater consequences this time. Who among us has not either fallen into a downward spiral or been afraid of following in my friend's footsteps? Who has not known the insatiable hunger of darkness?

"Lightness has a call that's hard to hear," but each time we choose to hear it, the call becomes a little clearer. We spend our days badgered by voices that tell us to judge others, fear others, harm others, or harm ourselves. But we are not obligated to listen to those voices, or even to take responsibility for them. They may be where we come from, but they are not where we are going. There is another voice, a voice that shines. *Ahimsa* is the practice of listening to that voice of lightness, cultivating that voice, trusting that voice, acting upon that voice.

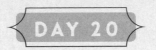

DAY 20

Free from all thoughts of "I" and "mine," that man finds utter peace.

Bhagavad Gita

As we begin to live the *yamas* and the *niyamas,* we make a joyful discovery. Having anticipated an onerous set of challenges and the not-too-distant prospect of failure, we arrive instead at an ancient truth: that to live according to these precepts is actually a relief. We realize that in fact these restraints and observances are in keeping with our own nature. We humans are meant to live in harmony, and the *yamas* and *niyamas* are simply a means to foster internal and external balance in our lives.

After writing an essay about *ahimsa,* I went to my local whole-foods store. I am a daily customer, and many of my students shop there as well, so I usually spend a good deal of time chatting with people I know. With the notion of nonharming so fresh in my mind, though, I found myself talking to people in the checkout line I did not know. The impulse to reach out came from the spiritual injunction at the heart of *ahimsa:* that we should not draw lines around ourselves, and that we should see all beings as our brothers and sisters. To my surprise that morning, I discovered that I enjoyed talking to strangers at least as much as I enjoyed talking to my friends and students.

Upon reflection, I realized that it was my own fear of rejection and my fear of others' judgment of me that had held me back from making this a regular practice. Many times I had experienced the joy and magic of connecting to strangers, but creating such connections had not become a habit, because of my own fear. As I've come to understand the true meaning of *ahimsa,* I've also found more connection with my world. With relief, I've begun to let go of my fear of other people. My fear of strangers has been an aspect of suffering in my life—and this *yama* challenges me to get over it. Our suffering is a reflection of imbalance and delusion; the *yamas* and *niyamas* bring us out of delusion, into clarity and balance. And with balance comes utter peace, and the joy we seek.

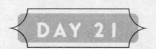

DAY 21

I learn by going where I have to go.

Theodore Roethke

I had breakfast the other morning with a woman who wants me to help her develop as a teacher. In an effort to be helpful, I asked a few questions about her life up to now. One of my questions was, "What has been hard?" She took a deep breath, then told me that a few years ago, when she was two months pregnant with her second child, she and her husband were told that there was something gravely wrong with the baby, but the doctors could not be certain what it was. The couple was told that abortion might be their best option. Instead, they decided to continue the pregnancy, and spent the next seven months in uncertainty. The baby was born healthy in every respect. She is now a beautiful, vibrant child. When they look upon her, her parents still recall those seven long months of faith and courage.

The truth is, we are all so very, very vulnerable. Life is as it is. We don't even have control over the health of our children. The only thing we *can* control is our attitude. We have the choice of life or death, love or fear, in each moment. And we bear the responsibility for that choice in each moment. Nowhere is this more apparent than when we embark on a regular yoga practice. We set out to be better ourselves, only to find legions of reasons to break our commitment to health. We say it is too difficult to make the hard choice today. And yet the obstacles in our path *are* the path. Every time we stretch beyond our resistance and our fear, we make a choice for life. And every time we choose life, we find that fear loses its grip on us. We all know more than we think we do, and we are stronger than we believe ourselves to be. We come to our mats, and to our lives, to learn by going where we have to go.

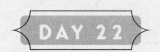

DAY 22

Ignorance creates all the other obstacles.

Yoga Sutras

A woman once told me that she loved travel because it offered her the opportunity to see how other people live. Her words stayed with me because, at the time, I was in the early years of my yoga practice and I honestly could not understand why anyone felt compelled to travel. In my early twenties I had spent years overseas with the military and had learned very little, because I was not really awake. Once I started yoga, everything about my practice seemed to be telling me that I could learn what I needed to know right here, right now. My problem, as I saw it, was that I had very little understanding of who I was or what I could be—or even what I wanted to be, for that matter.

My yoga practice was teaching me how to pay attention to my everyday life in a way that was beneficial to myself and those around me. I was getting a glimpse of the hugeness of the ordinary, the sacred beauty of the everyday. I felt I could spend a hundred lifetimes just refining my own ability to have a good day. To be able to move through the world in a manner that was in keeping with my values, and to be of service to myself and others, seemed like an enormous achievement. Why did I need to go anyplace in particular to do this? What made one patch of earth any more effective as a training ground than another?

I got my answer years later, when I took my wife on a vacation to Costa Rica. It is quite something to wake up in Cambridge, Massachusetts, on a frigid January morning and to go to bed that night in the jungle. Curiously, in Costa Rica I found that it is important to travel because leaving home offers us an opportunity to see how other people live. There were two lessons for me in this experience. First, we are able to hear only what we are ready to take in. As productivity guru David Allen points out, "Information is always available, but we are not always available to the information." Apparently I just wasn't ready to learn about the benefits of travel at the time of my conversation with my friend; I was deeply engaged in another sort of education, one that demanded all my energies right then. Of even more significance is the fact that we were both right. It is important to travel and it is also important to be here now.

Astanga yoga teacher and writer Beryl Bender Birch named her institute the Hard and the Soft in recognition that we all need both in our lives and in our practice. We need to acquire a win-win, "both"/"and" orientation. Yoga teaches us to develop open attention, attention without attachment or judgment. It was my judgment of this woman's view of the merits of travel that blocked my understanding and kept me in ignorance. Fortunately, it is also the nature of lessons to return to us until we understand them.

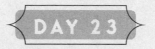

DAY 23

When the practitioner is firmly established in the practice of the truth, his words become so potent that whatever he says comes to realization.

Yoga Sutras

The first *yama, ahimsa,* concerns love, and the second, *satya,* concerns truth. *Satya* gives us our first experience of a paradox in yoga. We begin the practice of *satya* with considerable will and attention as we work hard to speak the truth and to live the truth. Every conversation, every mundane activity invites our scrutiny: are we being truthful in thought, word, and deed? Over time, though, the successful application of will and attention actually strips us of our need for both. Initially we experience *satya* as having to do with concrete events and words. Either we kept a commitment or we did not. Either we spoke truthfully or we did not. Little by little we notice, and then drop, our old habits of embellishment, obfuscation, minimization, self-aggrandizement, omission, rationalization, and exaggeration. The process calls on all our powers of self-control; we bring our will to bear on the practice of being truthful in all things. At first, then, *satya* is practiced from the outside in. Eventually, however, we become fully established in the practice of the truth—so much so that we begin to live *satya* from the inside out. As the layers of falsehood fall away, an intimacy develops with our own truth. Ultimately our truth becomes all there is. Truth becomes our essence and our reality, our deepest desire, and the air that we breathe.

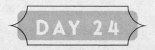

The only true currency in this bankrupt world is the truth that we share with one another when we are being uncool.

Line from the movie *Almost Famous*

This line from *Almost Famous* presents two profoundly beautiful and ordinary aspects of *satya:* letting go of pretense and telling the truth about ourselves to another human being. Haven't we all had those moments of startling honesty when we connected to the currency of sharing the truth without pretense—on a long bus ride with a stranger, perhaps, or under the stars on a summer night, or at the sickbed of a loved one, or every once in a while in therapy? These are holy moments, as we come out of hiding and allow ourselves to simply be truthful with another human being, without trying to be cool. As we come to see yoga playing at the edges of our lives, *satya* dancing across a movie screen, *ahimsa* (nonviolence) debated on the front page of the *New York Times,* we come to understand the idea of polytheism. We may attach all sorts of labels to our beliefs, and worship and practice in different ways. Yet we can recognize *satya* as a divine energy whose will is enacted in our lives individually and collectively. The power of the moment we share with a fine actor on the big screen was brought to us by the smiling goddess Satya.

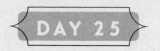

THE YAMAS

Pride goeth before destruction, and an haughty spirit
before a fall.

Proverbs 16:18

In practice, I often think of this proverb, and I remind my students, "Pride and ambition will get you hurt, humility will get you well." Putting *satya,* or truthfulness, into practice on the mat is an exercise in humility. We tend to vacillate between our pride and ambition and our fear. Think of a posture that you've almost nailed. You're so close to mastering it that you can almost taste it. How tempting it is to push now, to let your ego step in and take you the rest of the way. But when we become ambitious, we lose sight of the point of our practice.

Now think of a posture that you avoid. A student recently said she'd loved my class that morning. When I asked her what she had loved about it, she replied, "Well, we didn't do the crow." She speaks for all of us. I personally do not like the eagle pose. I have heavily muscled shoulders and heavily muscled thighs, and balancing on one leg with my arms and legs crossed over each other, I feel a lot more like the retired football player that I am than an eagle. When we avoid certain poses, though, we're allowing our own beliefs to dictate our reality. We believe that we are somehow less capable than the person to our right or to our left. The truth is that any demon honestly met becomes a friend, and our friends should be treated wisely if we wish them to remain our friends.

Instead of pride or ambition, fear or avoidance, we need the light of truth. Humility has two sides. Most of us have been told at one time or another, "Don't get too big for your breeches," and we know exactly what that means. Humility is about letting go of the good results as well as the bad. But there is another aspect to humility, and that is about not playing small. Just as we may strive on the mat for more than our bodies are ready for, we may also take the opposite tack, and play small. We back off and stay in the comfort zone, all our excuses at the ready: I'm not built like that; that's great for them but not for me; I have bad balance, bad knees, bad eyesight, the wrong kind of mat; it's too hot; it's too cold; I'm too young; I'm too old. We sell ourselves short.

Humility is also the awareness that we cannot afford to play small. It is the aspect of *satya* that brings us into balance. We need not eradicate fear or ambition; both are necessary energies in our lives. Rather, we must bring them into balance in the moment, so that our postures are practiced with a healthy distribution of both energies. Our postures become the embodiment of this exquisite balance between holding on and letting go, action and nonaction, ambition and restraint. What is required to achieve that balance is a commitment to humility, a commitment to the truth.

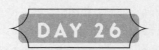

DAY 26

The real voyage of discovery consists not in seeking new landscapes, but in having new eyes.

Marcel Proust

We do not know what we do not know. Whenever I sit down to meditate or spend time on my mat, I am suddenly made conscious of the level of distraction in which I spend much of my time. I am writing these words the night before I am to fly to Mexico to teach a weeklong yoga retreat. To prepare myself, I've spent most of the day at a meditation center. There, as the quiet of prolonged meditation began to sink in, I slowly became aware of where I was coming from. In the course of the last week I've presided at my studio while we've been hosting a visiting teacher, undergoing major renovations, and introducing four new teachers into our schedule—all this while Boston was being pummeled by a three-day blizzard. I've also been making time to write each day, getting ready for the retreat, managing an unmanageable private class schedule, creating a new workshop format, teaching my regular classes, spending time with my wife and my dog, and doing my own yoga practice.

I did not experience this week as anything out of the ordinary because it is not. As I interacted with the visiting teacher, my new teachers, my students, the contractors, my wife, and my dog, I had no awareness of how much stress I was under—or of my responsibility for allowing that stress to be clouding my judgment. Finally, today, the utter stillness I found at the meditation center allowed me to arrive at an awareness that was not available to me all week as I rushed from one situation to the next. True, I was attending to my regular practice. But sometimes even that is not enough. There is power in regularly stepping back even further, going even deeper than we normally do. As we wade through the challenges, the opportunities, the joys, and the sorrows of our everyday lives, we must also honor our need to look upon our lives with new eyes. And the opportunity is always there. One morning spent in silence, an evening at a yoga workshop, an hour of quiet prayer in an empty church, an afternoon of meditation, or a weekend retreat—and we rediscover, reexperience, the truth of our lives and the roles we want to play in them.

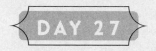

It is not because things are difficult that we do not dare; it is because we do not dare that they are difficult.

Seneca

The moment *satya* is brought up at a workshop, a heated discussion about truth always ensues. What if your partner comes downstairs wearing an unflattering new dress and asks what you think? Do you tell your boss he drives you nuts? Do you tell your employer about the padded expense account? And what about those sexual indiscretions that happened oh so long ago? Such ruminations are a staple in any discussion of the *yamas* and the *niyamas,* but they rarely bear fruit. It's my belief that they represent some sort of last-ditch ego effort to hold up the process. These protestations are the equivalent of the alcoholic's claim that she *would* stop drinking now, but since the holidays are coming up, it would be better to wait till next year; or the food addict's worries that if he gives up white sugar he won't be able to eat his wedding cake, despite the fact that he is recently divorced and not in a relationship.

Satya is about living our truth; it is that simple. There are as many ways to do this as there are people who practice *satya,* and no one can tell you how *you* should listen for and find the truth within yourself. It makes sense to talk things over with someone you trust, but the point of the discussion is to come closer to your truth, not to have someone relieve you of the responsibility of discerning your truth. For some of us it is a long road back to our own truth, for we live in a culture in which truth is a rare commodity. Our work environments, home lives, and friendships are often permeated with falsehood. We distrust the slogans of the media, the promises of our leaders, the testimonials of politicians, the declarations of business-people. Many of us come from families in which appearances are more important than reality. Still others have grown up in upside-down house-holds, in which children took care of parents or were expected to play pre-scribed roles in order to meet their parents' needs. Elaborate no-talk rules must be deconstructed. Old fears must be released. Habits of silence must be examined. Are we failing to speak the truth out of a desire to protect or care for others? How do we respond to information we know to be untrue? How do we get in touch with what is true and good within ourselves? The list of ways in which we have obscured the truth from ourselves and others is as endless as the suffering such obfuscation produces.

Before we begin this work, it can feel overwhelming. But we are each possessed of an inner compass. When we stand still in the wilderness and take our bearings, we are able to apprehend the truth—about ourselves and the world around us. And once we commence the practice of *satya,* we will never want to look back. We have only our own suffering to lose. As Plato said, "Truth is the beginning of every good thing, both in heaven and on earth; and he who would be blessed and happy should be from the first a partaker of truth, for then he can be trusted." Over time you will have the pleasure of watching this beautiful practice blossom in your life in a way that is honest and authentic. As you learn to speak the truth, you will learn to be true to yourself, to all that is best in you.

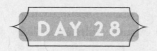

Nothing left. Isn't it something? Nothing left.

Pearl Jam

In Hindu thought there are four stages in the human journey. The first stage is the desire for pleasure, the second is the desire for success, the third is the desire for community, and the fourth is the desire for liberation. This progression is at once linear and nonlinear, for while they correspond to the different moments in a human life span, the four stages are also occurring all at once in every moment of our lives. The concept of these evolutionary stages is particularly useful to me, as a yoga teacher living in the United States in the twenty-first century, because yoga is about getting unstuck—and our society is currently stuck in the search for success.

Many students come to yoga having moved through the desire for success and having discovered a yearning for something larger—a spiritual connection, a sense of community. Others arrive at my studio still immersed in their quest for success, only to find that yoga connects them to these deeper spiritual longings. To move forward, then, into the next stage of the human journey, we must break with the past.

This is not a small thing. Our need to succeed is tied into the expectations of our families, gender, class, society, the whole enchilada. Under normal circumstances, letting go of our own self-image as an achiever, as a winner in the game of life, is a difficult transition. It is nothing less than the death of one self and the birth of another. For many Americans, stuck as we are in our cult of youthful ambition, this break feels akin to an act of treason. In our culture, the normal process of spiritual maturation recognized by the Hindus appears to be a denial of all that is sacred. Are we now to become New Age poseurs, masking our inability to fight the good fight with "spiritual" platitudes about "taking care of ourselves"? And if this change is necessary and even desirable, how are we to reconcile our new priorities with all those years sacrificed on the altar of success? My studio is one of the many stages on which this dilemma is playing itself out in this country. And I am but one of many witnesses to the drama.

We all get stuck somewhere along the path. The good news is that eventually we find that we have no choice but to let go and move on. We may temporize, rationalize, attempt to compromise. We may denounce the system, we may even grieve. But finally we do begin to grow again. When my older sister died I fought against the loss for years. Even as I mourned her death, I railed against the injustice of it—she was too young, too bright, too full of promise and possibility to die.

At long last I came to the breakthrough point, the surrender. I realized that her life, and my fury, were truly over. She was gone, and if I really loved her, I owed it to her to ensure that her passing would bear spiritual fruit in my life. For that to happen, I would have to let go. The relief was profound. There was nothing left to do.

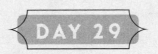

DAY 29

Those forms of concentration which result in extraordinary perceptions encourage perseverance of mind.

Yoga Sutras

Those on a spiritual path often say that we get what we need, not what we want. This statement can be viewed in a dim light. "Oh great," we think, "I'll have this humble, drab life because that's what I *need,* while all my friends are enjoying beautiful lives."

Experience has taught me that a good life is available to each one of us. If you were to write down everything you really want to have in your life five years from now, and if you were to persist in your spiritual practice in the interim, I suspect that at the end of the five years, you would find you had actually sold yourself short, because in truth, what the universe has in store for each of us is so much greater than anything we can imagine for ourselves.

So why are we so shortsighted? For one thing, most of us glimpse little of our real potential. If we knew who we really were, there would be no need for practices like yoga. It is our nature to see ourselves only in part, "as in a glass, darkly," but not whole. We may know those around us better than they know themselves, but it is our fate to know only a little about ourselves. For many of us, the first step toward health is realizing that we don't always know what is best for us.

Our imaginations are also limited by our inability to grasp the full effects of spiritual practice. By spiritual practice I don't mean doing yoga postures or sitting on a meditation pillow. I mean right action, walking the walk day in and day out. The truth is, a single right action has a tremendously positive effect—and a series of interconnected right actions will cause your life to become unrecognizable in a hurry. We see this all around us. Think of that enviable, perfect friend who doesn't seem to work at a spiritual practice, who is already sweet and loving, and who always does the right thing. Perhaps her life seems charmed; she appears to float along swimmingly as obstacles fall away before her. But in reality, this friend is doing the work all the time; she has learned to take right action as a matter of course. And doing the work encourages perseverance of mind because, ultimately, doing the work feels a lot better than dodging it.

As we take right action—as we pay the bill, delay the gratification, make the tough phone call, take the vacation, don't take the vacation, say yes, say no, show up for life—we accrue more energy. And each right action infuses us with the energy and the ability to take the next right action.

Thus we may cultivate the powers of concentration and remove
the obstacles to enlightenment which cause all our sufferings.

Yoga Sutras

As far as I know, my feet have been flat all my life. As a young person I was told I was very good at physical things, so I assumed that everything about my body was superlative, including my feet. Later, as an adolescent and then in my early twenties, I was involved in activities that seemed far more important than my feet, so I didn't assume anything about them. As I approached thirty, though, I no longer thought of my body as exceptional, nor did I find my life quite so compelling, either. I was ready for yoga.

Oddly, my yoga teacher didn't think my feet were ready for yoga. Not only were my feet flat, she said, but they represented a character flaw. She claimed that my feet weren't really flat, they were just lazy, and I needed to learn to lift my arches. I looked at her dumbly, then stared down at my feet. There they were, just where I had left them. I began to see her point—they *were* flat! If I was really going to practice yoga, my teacher patiently explained, I would have to figure out how to lift my arches when I was in standing postures. At first this made as much sense to me as willing my teeth to bend, but she assured me it was possible. I gave it a try. My toes turned out to be quite responsive. They lifted enthusiastically when asked, and even spread a little, once I sent them the message that that was what they were supposed to do.

The effort to establish a relationship with my toes laid the groundwork for my next frontier, the bottoms of my feet. Six months of intensive toe lifting, spreading, and gripping had a remarkable effect on the soles of my feet. They were stronger, more alive. The bottoms of my feet had developed so profoundly that I was now walking on a cushion of foot muscle! My confidence soared, and so did my arches. Equipped with active toes and buff foot bottoms, I was finally able to activate my arches—easily.

Now hardly a day goes by that I don't lift my arches with pleasure. My feet provide a stable platform for my practice and for my life. In fact, my entire skeletal system has undergone a restructuring. In the course of regular practice, I have corrected a significant case of scoliosis and, in the process, ended fifteen years of back pain. My experience is not unique. Through yoga, we learn to bring our attention to a particular area in our bodies, or in our lives, and keep it there—and the results are nothing short of miraculous. The only thing that seems certain is that we cannot imagine the power of a mind, a will, and a body refined by yoga. We must experience such transformation for ourselves.

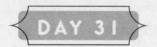

DAY 31

When abstention from stealing is firmly established, precious jewels come.

Yoga Sutras

The third *yama* is *asteya,* or nonstealing. *Asteya* serves as a wake-up call, prompting us to remember all the ways, big and small, that we steal—the borrowed books still on our shelves, the corners we cut on our taxes, the hours we spend at work not being productive. As we begin to consciously practice *asteya,* we also see just where and how we need to change. Suddenly we are no longer comfortable with the rationalizations and compromises we have been making.

At a deeper level, *asteya* is our first encounter with the power of nonattachment. When we look honestly at the ways in which we have been steal-ing, we come to understand that in each instance, there is an attachment to a specific result that overrides our deeper values. We want the last orange in the refrigerator more than we want to be a good partner. We had a tough week at work, so we will undertip the waitress at the diner. Beneath the attachment, we find fear: fear that we will not get what we need; fear that if we leave things up to the universe, we will not be taken care of. This sutra declares the opposite to be true: "When abstention from stealing is firmly established, precious jewels come." In other words, the surest way to get what you want is to let go of wanting. What is required, then, is a radical, absolute, living trust in the workings of the universe. This trust is the spiri-tual opposite of the act of stealing, and accompanied by right action, it removes the blocks to our natural abundance.

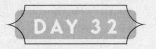

The kingdom of heaven is like a merchant in search of fine
pearls, who, on finding one pearl of great value, went and sold
all that he had and bought it.

Matthew 13:45

In this New Testament statement on the nature of enlightenment, we see again the fundamental truth and power behind *asteya,* or nonstealing. *Asteya* presents us with an opportunity to put our faith into action. Are we willing to give up all we have for the pearl that is our spiritual growth? For most of us the answer is, "Not yet." *Asteya* serves as a mirror, revealing ourselves to ourselves. As we shine the spotlight of our awareness on nonstealing, we begin to see the manifold ways in which we act out faithlessness instead of faith.

I've just returned from teaching at a weeklong yoga retreat on a remote beach in Mexico. It was the most powerful experience of that sort I have ever had. I was either practicing yoga, teaching yoga, meditating, chanting, or fasting for seven straight days. The closing ceremony was deeply moving, as the sixty-five participants shared their personal stories of healing and transformation. The next morning, I borrowed a pair of scissors from the hotel staff and began to remove the inspirational quotes we had posted on the walls of the yoga studio. As I used the scissors, I realized that they would be helpful on the next retreat, which was only three weeks away and at the same facility. So I wisely stored the scissors in my bag with the quotes.

As I went to check out, the manager of the hotel asked me about the scissors. We were in the jungle, a few miles from town, and scissors apparently do not grow on trees down there. So I had the good fortune of opening up my suitcase in front of this loving woman to retrieve her scissors. This in the midst of my writing on *asteya*. Be careful what you pray for.

My attempted theft of this woman's scissors gave me pause to think. It certainly brought home to me the difference between doing a lot of spiritual practice and truly standing in my spirituality. An Alcoholics Anonymous text says, "Either God is or he is not." Each theft, each time we "forget" to return something we've borrowed, each moment we give in to the impulse to covet or to be jealous, we are saying, "My God is not." To practice *asteya,* we must abandon ourselves to the care of the universe. We must be willing to give up all we have for the one true thing. We must say in each moment, with each thought, word, and deed, "My God is."

They who in every least thing are wholly honest with the spirit
of life, find life supporting them in all things.

Charles Johnston

The initial work we do on *asteya,* or nonstealing, concerns outright acts of theft. To our surprise, most of us find there is significant work to do. Each of the *yamas* is an excercise in faith; as we work with them, we put our faith into action. Nonstealing on the physical plain is really about believing that the universe will take care of our needs, and acting accordingly. This is a very powerful thing to do. As we deepen this work, we discover our willingness to take the next step, to examine our habitual thoughts, attitudes, and beliefs.

In the previous essay I confessed to my attempted theft of a pair of scissors. Behind this transgression, of course, was my own unexamined belief in scarcity. I felt that it was prudent to take the scissors because everybody knows that life is chaotic and you can't always get what you need when you need it. When you do get something you need, you had better hold on to it. Without too much effort, I had myself convinced that I was being wise in the ways of the world, and I told myself I was actually acting on the fruits of hard-earned experience. And the universe said, "Wrong! Thanks for playing. Now give the scissors back to the nice lady and try it again."

Until we begin to acknowledge the poverty consciousness that drives us to steal—to commit those tiny, seemingly insignificant thefts without a second thought—we cannot significantly change our behavior. *Asteya* is our opportunity to let go of poverty consciousness. We no longer have to believe that if *you* win, *I* lose. We no longer have to defend our opinions, or anything else for that matter. We can begin to live in harmony with the flow of life. We find that we have been like salmon who, mistaking ourselves for beaver, have vigorously set about damming the river and making lodges. Despite the fact that we find this extremely difficult without beaver teeth and beaver paws, we spend a lifetime working to create the perfect beaver pond. Then an enlightened salmon comes along and explains that the river will take us effortlessly out to the ocean—where we belong and where we will grow into our full salmonhood. We are told that the river we have spent so much energy blocking and hoarding is actually endless and will deliver us to a place of unimaginable abundance. All that is required is for us to stop blocking the flow with our misguided efforts, our misguided beliefs.

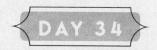

DAY 34

Our vision is beclouded and the pathway of our progress is
obstructed until we come to know that God can and does
express as Good in every person and every situation.

Ernest Holmes

Students approach me after class with two sorts of problems. Some have nagging physical difficulties or have injured themselves while exercising or playing sports. Others have emotional injuries. They may be going through a divorce, be out of work or stuck in their careers, or suffer from anxiety or depression; or they may just have difficult lives and feel sad. Having experienced most of these troubles myself, and professing no expertise in anything, all I can offer is compassion, as I explain how I meet my own hardships. Over time I've been struck by the fact that as I get progressively more honest, what I have to say becomes progressively more simple.

A physical problem that affects us on the mat is an opportunity to pay closer attention to what we do, and to put our faith in our ability to heal. A life problem off the mat, whether it has to do with the IRS or childhood abuse, is an opportunity to pay closer attention to what we do, and to put our faith in our ability to heal.

There was a time when I used the word "mindfulness," suggesting that these situations were opportunities to develop mindfulness. But I've since felt the need to break that word down. A person in pain often needs things to be broken down. Mindfulness is the art of paying attention. But there is more to it than that. It is paying attention with an abiding faith in a loving universe. We are not meant to be on the edge of our seats, anxiously paying attention so that we can control outcomes and events. We are meant to stand firmly in the postures of our lives, bearing witness to the moment, to our experience of the moment, aware as we do so that, in the words of Charles Johnston, "we are encompassed and supported by spiritual powers." When we pay attention with faith that we will be supported, then growth really is possible, our vision becomes clear, our path becomes unobstructed, and we are able to see the "Good in every person and situation."

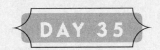

DAY 35

The posture never ends.

Rolf Gates

I teach a flowing style of yoga in which one posture flows into the next. The transitions between postures are postures in their own right. The breath and the meditation are unbroken. This is not true in all styles of yoga, nor is such a flow necessary in order for a form of yoga to be effective. The lesson remains, however, that it is our tendency to pay attention to the postures themselves, but not to the spaces in between. So it is in life. We leave one relationship or job and set our sights on the next. We cross one item off the to-do list and dive into the next chore. The illusion is that the posture ends. The reality is that the posture never ends, it just shifts from one form to the next, one lesson to the next, one opportunity to the next. We remain life's student whether we are inhaling or exhaling, in a relationship or out of one, saving the world or looking for a temp job. The posture never ends. I am in the posture when I look into my wife's eyes, and I am in the posture when I look into my waiter's eyes. Both are holy interactions. The illusion is that there is separation, levels of importance, beginnings and endings. Yoga brings us to the understanding that the posture never ends.

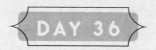

On these sands and in the clefts of the rocks, in the depths of the sea, in the creaking of the pines, you'll spy secret footprints and catch far-off voices from the homecoming celebration. This land still longs for Odysseus.

Homer

I am struck by the pervasive desire for homecoming in this passage, an ancient, secret longing. Here is a sadness and an emptiness so profound that it is felt by rocks and trees. It is in the air—a sadness that is bittersweet because it is a reminder of better days, an innocence lost. Before yoga, each of us is like the land that longs for the return of its hero. We can feel this

PART ONE

The Beginning

longing in our muscles, in our bones, in the movements that were once fluid and natural but that have become prematurely stiff and unreliable. There is a presence, a life force, that is conspicuous in its absence. But over time, this sense of loss becomes just another aspect of the subtly shifting backdrop of our lives. Yes, we were once possessed of a youthful vitality, but many of us forgot we ever had such vigor and energy long before we came to our first yoga class. And then the moment of homecoming arrives. Unbidden, unsought—we hear the familiar footsteps on the porch. For me it occurred at the end of one of my first classes. I was in a knee-down twist, moments before *shavasana*. I don't remember the rest of the class, but I do remember a sudden opening and a sense of suppleness in my spine that I'd never expected to experience again. I felt well in a way that I had let go of ever wanting to feel again.

There is a wisdom within us that is more powerful than our despair. There is a movement toward health that our intellect can merely glimpse, once in a while. It is the same impulse that causes plants to face the sun, animals to take care of their young, people who say, "I never sweat," to try a hot yoga class. This life force has provided us with the priceless, miraculous opportunity of our yoga practice. All we need to do is cultivate an open heart, to express our gratitude both on and off the mat, and to celebrate the return of our hero.

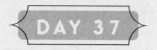

When the practitioner is firmly established in continence, knowledge, vigor, valor, and energy flow to him.

Yoga Sutras

The fourth *yama* is the discipline of *brahmacarya,* which literally means to "walk with God." Although it is often translated as "chastity," *brahmacarya* also means "continence." It is, quite simply, a call for us to practice moderation. The arena most associated with *brahmacarya* is sexuality, and this *yama* is often misunderstood as the expectation that we be celibate, on the assumption that the celibate yogi is somehow more enlightened. This is definitely not the point. B. K. S. Iyengar, in his discussion of *brahmacarya,* points out that the yogi Vasistha had one hundred children and yet was still living within the definition of *brahmacarya.* To focus on celibacy is to miss the power of the final *yama* altogether. *Brahmacarya* is not a call for abstinence but a call for temperance. As we practice *brahmacarya,* we have the opportunity to enact the balance that is yoga in all that we do. We can bring moderations to our thoughts, words, and deeds.

We live in a world that is decidedly intemperate. Since the Industrial Revolution the operative word in American culture has been "more." I recently received a phone call letting me know that I had been preapproved for a credit card with a $30,000 line of credit. Having carried a $4,000 plastic debt over a period of five or six impoverished years immediately after leaving the service, I considered $20,000 or $30,000 of credit card debt growing at a cyclic rate to be the stuff of my nightmares. But this offer is typical of the invitations to self-destructive immoderation that bombard all of us every day. Entreaties for us to conserve, to reuse, and to live simply are but a drop in the vast ocean of "More!" *Brahmacarya* offers us a chance to resist the culture of overindulgence and to bring a spirit of temperance into our lives.

Practicing *brahmacarya* is quite simple, and the results are immediate. The Yoga Sutras tells us that valor, vigor, knowledge, and energy flow to those who practice moderation. A quick inventory will illuminate how we are doing in a given area. Does my sex life fill me with valor, vigor, knowledge, and energy? Or is it a cause for concern, anxiety, confusion, and stress? How about food? Am I energized by my food, or obsessed by it? Do I feel liberated by the choices that I make around my food, or am I filled with concern, anxiety, and stress? We can go on to examine our relationships with money, work, time management, hobbies, exercise—whatever preoccupies our days. As we consider these questions honestly, it becomes easy to see where we are being intemperate and how the first small steps into moderation can be life changing.

Brahmacarya is the feeling of freedom that comes when we have let an addictive craving go—when we can eat to live, not live to eat; when we can work to live, not live to work; when we stand firmly and with ease of heart in the postures of life.

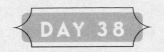

DAY 38

I listen to the wind, to the wind of my soul.

Cat Stevens

Brahmacarya, or temperance, gets a very bad rap in our culture. Most of us associate moderation with repression. The hero of the story loves the fair maiden, loves her passionately, and then the repressive forces come in to wreck the day. No one ever seems to dedicate poems, screenplays, or odes to the joys of moderation or the rewards of passionate balance. As a species we seem unable to see the forest for the trees. Despite the staggering amount of evidence that excess destroys our dreams, there appears to be a human blind spot when it comes to the possibility that our most passionate existence might actually be accessed through balance and moderation. Once we actually start to bring *brahmacarya* into our lives, we find that this *yama* is about truly following one's heart. We see that the chaos of immoderation brings us pain and anguish—and that the calm, clear energy released by moderation actually affords us the opportunity to realize all our dreams.

The moment I fall off the moderation wagon, my mind becomes consumed by the fact that I am no longer living up to my potential. My mind fills with obsessive concern; I know all too well the ways I am self-sabotaging. My heart yearns for peace. Then I wake up one morning and find that I have made a decision. I am ready to let go of whatever it is that's consuming me. I am ready to reestablish *brahmacarya* in my life. I am ready to follow my heart. I am ready to listen to the wind of my soul.

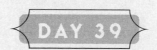

DAY 39

If you haven't heard from him, it just means you didn't call.

Van Morrison

Yesterday I wrote about waking up one morning and being ready to let go of what had been consuming me. Perhaps you thought, "Well, that sounds great, but how did you get to that point?" Any discussion of *vairagya* (renunciation) or *brahmacarya* (moderation) necessarily leads to a discussion of prayer. This is a book about yoga, not prayer, and yet I feel it's important to point out that prayer is the original spiritual practice. Long after all our other practices have fallen by the wayside, and no matter how much pain we are in or how self-destructive we have been, prayer is available to us. And prayer will find us the energy we need to come back from the brink. The message of the Buddha, of Christ, and of yoga is the possibility of resurrection, redemption, rebirth. Prayer is the locomotive that drives the resurrection train.

If we are to seriously consider enacting all of the *yamas* and *niyamas* in our lives, we must begin to examine the idea of spiritual force, spiritual momentum. Any honest individual will admit that to truly live the *yamas* and *niyamas* would require a radical shift. In fact, to make the realization of all the *yamas* and *niyamas* your aim in life is to desire the impossible. But prayer makes the impossible possible. Prayer enables us to tap into the healing power of the universe. We do not *do* the *yamas* and *niyamas;* we allow them to be enacted through us. We allow their energies to flourish in the world through us as we surrender to them. Prayer is the means by which we formally surrender. Going to the mat is a form of surrender; abstaining from violence and being truthful are forms of surrender. Prayer *is* surrender. The simplest prayer I know is "Thy will be done." The next simplest is "Please help me with . . ." When praying, it helps to keep things simple and selfless. If you don't know who you are praying *to,* join the club—no one does, for sure. If you meet someone who does know, read his or her book. In the meantime, be a yogi and experiment to find out what works for you. Whenever I pray, things have a way of working out far better than I could imagine. This has so often been true that it brings me to tears thinking that there are people whose fears will not allow them to receive the beauty that prayer has brought into my life. Let the power of prayer speak for itself. And if you haven't heard from the spirit of the universe, that just means you haven't called.

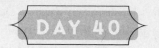

DAY 40

Do right, fear no man.
Dan Capel, U.S. Navy SEAL

All the translations of the Yoga Sutras I come across link *brahmacarya,* or moderation, with courage. The connection makes sense when we consider the state of intemperance. Nothing is more debilitating than the dread associated with immoderation in any area of our lives. The state of active addiction is accompanied by an overwhelming sense of impending doom. Even in less extreme situations, that fear is profoundly destructive to our belief in ourselves.

At the core of intemperance in any form is the mistaken belief that we are not OK as we are. Convinced that we are imperfect, we carry real pain. The cause of our suffering, however, is not our imperfection but our mistaken belief in our imperfection. Acting under the erroneous assumption that we are imperfect, we reach outside ourselves to create balance, to end our suffering. Naturally this is unsuccessful, so we redouble our efforts and demand even more. All our effort, all our striving, merely worsens our situation and deepens our conviction that we are somehow flawed. Caught up in this cycle of chronic suffering and misguided attempts to relieve our pain, we spend our days out of balance and in conflict with ourselves.

The solution is twofold. To begin with, we have to stop whatever it is we are doing that creates imbalance. When you are stuck in a hole, stop digging. The second step is to examine the beliefs that drive us to intemperance in the first place. *Brahmacarya* concerns the first step, summoning the courage to step away from the downward spiral. We discover that there is a power in nondoing. As we practice moderation, a wind begins to fill our sails. We find that the ever-present anxiety that accompanies immoderation evaporates. We realize that our fear, which grew out of a specific behavior, had contaminated every aspect of our lives. And as we finally walk away from the food, the sex, the alcohol, the debt, the fill-in-the-blank, we leave our fear behind as well. Suddenly we can begin to meet people's eyes again. We are no longer making up excuses for our reality. The colors of our lives become brighter and bolder. We find that when we do right, we fear no man.

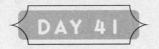

DAY 41

Let us never negotiate out of fear,
but let us never fear to negotiate.

John F. Kennedy

Brahmacarya on the mat is suppleness of spirit. As we return to our mats over and over again, we experience rigidity at many levels. We can become rigidly attached to practicing at certain times, certain temperatures, in certain styles, certain sequences, with certain teachers, certain clothes, certain mats, certain places in the room, certain towels, certain results . . . The list is endless. Many of these attachments are harmless. Most of us settle down to a particular style and a particular philosophy, and this is necessary if we are to dig our wells deep. Nevertheless, the root of all attachment is fear, and a fear-driven practice gets us hurt or gets us nowhere at all. *Brahmacarya* on the mat is the sensitivity to these attachments. Where and in what manner am I out of balance? Am I practicing seven days a week to control my weight, or to achieve a body shape I believe will give me power in the world? Am I practicing yoga as a means to show up for my life, or to hide from it? Do I appreciate my teacher because she challenges me to look at my life, or because she doesn't make me look at my life? As we cultivate this sort of inquiry on the mat, our practice becomes an exercise in balance.

As a rule of thumb in my own practice, I avoid becoming complacent. That means two things: I rest more often than I like, and I take class even when I don't want to. I believe that it's good for me to be pushed harder than I would like, and that it's equally good for me to take time off, or to practice without pushing at all. I know that if I don't like a teacher, it's because she reflects an aspect of myself that I have not made peace with. I know that I will never graduate, and I know, too, that I can trust my body. *Brahmacarya* on the mat is the same as it is anywhere else—it is Sanskrit for personal responsibility.

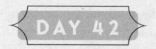

DAY 42

Karma is the eternal assertion of human freedom. . . .
Our thoughts, our words, and deeds are threads of the net
we throw around ourselves.

Swami Vivekananda

As we go deeper into the practice of *brahmacarya,* we connect to one of the underpinnings of yoga—the law of karma. Every science student knows the Newtonian concept that every action causes an equal and opposite reaction. Karma works the same way: what goes around comes around; whatever we put out into the world comes back onto us. Imagine that each one of us lives at the center of a spider's web of his or her own making. The threads of the web are our thoughts, words, and deeds; all together, these strands form our karma. Yoga is the conscious manipulation of karma. It is the study of how to avoid injurious karma and how to accrue positive karma. The ultimate aim of yoga is to transcend this web of karma, so that we can reunite with our divinity.

Brahmacarya gives us an excellent opportunity to see the law of karma in action. There is the middle road, and while on it we experience "knowledge, vigor, valor, and energy." If we indulge in immoderation, though, even for a moment, we immediately embark on another set of experiences—namely, guilt, remorse, obsessive worry, inertia. It is really that simple. We all the know the price of eating too much, spending too much, drinking too much—a few minutes of pleasure, followed by hours of guilt and remorse. When we choose to stay on the middle road, though, we experience a sense of well-being. On the middle road I am free; in immoderation I am compromised, sidetracked, shackled to negative self-talk. As we experience these lessons, we begin to learn the extent to which the choices that we make affect our inner world. We begin to see that the only peace to be found comes through moderation. We eventually understand the hand we play in creating the world we live in. We begin to see that karma is not an oppressive hand of fate; rather, it is the "eternal assertion" that we are free.

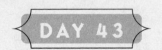

DAY 43

Whether you and I and a few others will renew the world
some day remains to be seen. But within ourselves we must
renew it each day.

Hermann Hesse

Two months ago, responding in part to the inspiration of living and writing this book, I returned to a more moderate relationship to food. In the ensuing transformation, I've rediscovered a younger, lighter, more beautiful body. My practice has become more precise and gentle. I actually feel a feminine grace in my body, as if I'm becoming soft, light, and pretty. Now, it is important to remember that I am a 175-pound ex-wrestler and football player, and so all of these adjectives are relative. Nevertheless, they accurately describe my experience of my new body.

Sitting in a cab on my way home from the airport the other night, with my newly supple hips conforming lightly to the backseat, I suddenly understood a clinical truth that I had known intellectually for quite some time: that many obese people find their efforts to lose weight thwarted because, as they return to a healthy weight, they also return to their former selves— to smaller selves, selves that were vulnerable in ways they found intolerable. At some unconscious level, the pain of obesity can be preferable to the pain of reexperiencing those old selves, and so the weight begins to come back on. As I sat in the cab late at night, riding through Boston, the city of my adolescence, I felt once again all the youthful concerns I'd harbored about being soft and light and pretty. And I understood for the first time, at a gut level, why we try to protect ourselves with layers of armor, why we clothe our youthful, defenseless selves with bulk or fat or muscle, in a subconscious attempt to arm ourselves against the world.

Progress in the practice of yoga postures de-ages us, peeling away the years. Stretching, strengthening, moving our bodies, we travel back in time, moving through a series of former selves. As we continue in our practice, we have an opportunity to resolve many of the issues we were incapable of resolving at earlier moments in our lives. The process can be exhilarating, but it can also be harrowing, difficult, and destabilizing. Our bodies hold our memories deep within, and yoga brings them to the fore once again.

Ours is a specifically physical spiritual discipline. It is about the body. We live in a culture that profits from our fears and negative beliefs about our bodies, and many of us have internalized that negativity. As we embrace our physical discipline, we come face-to-face with all our negative beliefs and images, a lifetime's worth, in fact. But these images are not who we are. Our practice, and the resulting transformation, affords us the opportunity to let go. As we begin to really live in our bodies and experience our true power, we are also able to move on, to put aside that which is no longer ours.

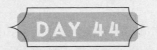

DAY 44

What is the key to untie the knot of your mind's suffering?
Act great. My dear, always act great.

Hafez

I recently met with my new accountant. For days I looked forward to this event, fantasizing that I would be able to hand all my financial matters over to him, thereby freeing myself to move on to more spiritual concerns. Instead, he asked me to do some homework and get back to him within a week. It took me five weeks. First there was my vacation, then there was all the work waiting for me when I got back, and finally there was the gnawing sense that with each passing week, my fantasy of financial freedom was turning into a nightmare. Eventually I decided to heed my own advice, and take the right action. Embarrassed and sheepish, I sent off my information and continued my movement toward financial health.

The eight-limb path is all about behavior. It's about our actions, not our good intentions. If we want self-esteem, we must do estimable things. The emphasis is on the doing. Hafez, a fourteenth-century Sufi poet, suggests that we act great all the time. He doesn't suggest that we wait around until we feel good and then, with the necessary "feeling-good" momentum, begin acting great. He urges us to act great whether we feel good or not. And short of that ideal, we ought to fake it until we make it.

This advice holds true for all the practices of this path. Whether we are practicing contentment on a bad day, muddling through the first yoga class of our lives, or are sitting in meditation watching our mind run around in circles, the key is the same: just do it. If you want to be graceful in your movements, don't listen to the negative self-talk. Instead, act *as if*. Take up space, be grand, act great. Move with exaggerated grace and precision, and before long your body will get with the program. If you want to meditate, staple your butt to the cushion; sooner or later your mind will quiet down. If you want to practice moderation, spend less, eat more slowly, take your to-do list and cut it in half, make a beginning. We can count on the new and the unfamiliar to be awkward. But the awkwardness of that first step is no reason for us to deny ourselves the opportunity to have balance in a given area of our lives. We will have the degree of grace in our lives that we permit ourselves to have.

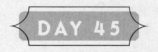

DAY 45

The prize is in the process.
Baron Baptiste

One day after class a woman came to me to ask about her practice. She said she was finding that a good challenging practice every other day was not working for her, because she wasn't experiencing the progress she wanted. As her story unfolded, it was clear that she liked the "wow" feeling of tangible progress in her postures, and that she was also concerned about the appearance of her postures because she was considering teaching yoga herself.

This student's concerns bring up a couple of common challenges. How often should we practice? It might well be that this woman's body would be better-served by practicing five or six days a week, and I suggested that she experiment with practicing more often, with an eye for symptoms of over-training. But all of us must work out for ourselves what is the right amount of time to spend doing asana. And this will change from week to week, from life moment to life moment, as other demands on our time and energy wax and wane.

The next part of her question concerned attachment. In this case, it was attachment to progress, to the exhilaration of physical breakthroughs, and to specific results. Unfortunately, the reasonable desire for ego-gratifying results must be abandoned in yoga. If we are really practicing yoga and abiding by the principals of yoga, then we are making a commitment to focus on the nature of our efforts and not the nature of the results. The sort of attachment to progress this student describes is not only antithetical to the true aim of yoga, it is also a one-way ticket to injury and burnout. When we focus on what we can get out of yoga, we miss the point. We also place ourselves in physical danger while sabotaging our relationship to our practice. To realize the beauty of yoga in our lives, we must never forget that the prize is in the process.

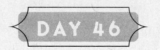

The cracked vase lasts.

Anonymous

I was driving around town one morning, full of conflict, having arguments with people who weren't there—and I was winning. A police car's flashing lights jolted me out of my reverie, and a moment later I received a ticket for driving with an expired inspection sticker. I went through my usual drill for when bad things happen to good people—practiced letting go and all that—and went home. A few days later, I found myself engaged in another conflict and spending hours obsessing about it. This time, though, I paused to notice that as I put my energies into stewing, my responsibilities faded into the background. Caught up in the emotions of my latest conflict, I had lost touch with the realities of my life. I realized that conflict, for me, has the potential of being a place I go when I should be living in reality instead. One of the responsibilities I had yet to take care of was getting my car inspected. The violation-dispensing policeman had been a messenger from reality, asking me to come home.

In yoga, injuries often stand in for the reality police. There are as many different reasons for injury in yoga as there are people who practice yoga, and it is possible for an injury to have no particular message. My personal experience, however, and the experience of every student who has ever discussed an injury with me, suggests that injuries don't happen in a vacuum. In fact, injuries are part of the interconnected web of our mind, body, spirit, and relationships. More often than not, injuries are lessons.

I developed a minor form of tendonitis in my elbow while learning astanga's primary series. I had had tendonitis in that elbow from riding a bike on city streets for years, and so it was tempting to say that this was simply an old injury rearing its head again. But as I analyzed my yoga I had to admit to myself that there was a lot of impatience and thoughtlessness in my transition from *chaturanga* to upward dog. In astanga yoga, you make that transition innumerable times in the course of a two-hour practice, and I was getting bored and sloppy. Just as, moments before being pulled over in the car, I had been lost in my thoughts and could not have been further from reality, I was now drifting away in my practice when I should have been fully present. I was not paying attention to the movement required to bring my body forward and up with grace. The tendonitis in my elbow was an invitation to return to reality.

This is not to say that we deserve our injuries, or even that all injuries are the result of distraction or sloppy work. But our injuries do offer us an opportunity to pay attention. When we accept the invitation and bring our awareness to the root causes of an injury and to the work required to heal, we invariably find that we've moved into a deeper level of practice as a result. Our greatest liability can become our greatest asset.

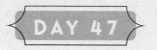

DAY 47

It is high time now that we should return to the plainness and
soundness of observations on material and obvious things.

Robert Hooke

Watching the Oscars this year, I could not help but reflect that the essence of all spiritual teachings was right before our eyes. The message could not have been plainer or more obvious. Here we have arguably the most beautiful and powerful people on earth, resplendent in beauty and attire, intoxicating in their ability to control events and gain desired outcomes. These are the individuals who embody our most treasured visions of worldly power and success . . . But wait—isn't that So-and-so, who was so popular three years ago? Isn't that So-and-so, who is going through a nasty divorce and hasn't had a good movie in years? And look at So-and-so, so beautiful, so powerful, so happy receiving today's Oscar from last year's winner. And what about last year's winner? He looks older, maybe a little less happy, a little less special. What has he done lately? And doesn't it show in the lackluster way he holds himself? Where is the confidence of last year? Where are the signs that this man—so powerful, so capable—has the degree of control over events that we so ardently strive for? Is it possible that the control we yearn for is not part of the deal?

When a Roman general returned in triumph to the Eternal City, the multitudes turned out and he was feted as he rode through the streets to the Capitol. But at his ear was a servant who whispered, "Glory is fleeting." The signs of our impermanence are all around us, yet we continue to hold out hope that someday, somehow, we will receive a different message. Those of us who follow sports remember that the Chicago Bulls of the mid-nineties were immortal. Their accomplishments defied comparison—but where are they now? Who can make life stop in its tracks, or turn back the hands of time? Yet our yearnings for something larger than life, for something eternal to believe in, are not inappropriate; they are simply misguided.

At two points during the Oscar ceremony we caught a glimpse of real greatness, of the human capacity to endure the ravages of time. There were two lifetime achievement awards, given out by friends to their mentors. The recipients of these awards were both in their eighties, having spent their entire lives in the movie industry. As they reflected on the nature of their accomplishments, they did not list their accolades or triumphs. Instead, they spoke of the passionate love they had for their art and of the joy they felt at having been able to be of service. In the Bhagavad Gita we are told that we transcend our suffering to the degree that we are able to passionately employ our gifts in the service of others. As these men approach the end of their lives, this seems to be what they are telling us as well.

PART ONE
The Beginning
1

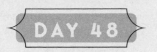

**It is always 3 A.M., raining, and you are at the intersection of
two maps, when your country needs you the most.**

U.S. military officers' joke

Although I heard this line countless times in the army, and although it isn't true, I still got the message: the only way to ensure that you will never find yourself in this predicament is to be prepared for it. In that sense, this bit of institutional army wisdom was helpful to me, for I heeded it as a warning. And I couldn't help but be reassured by the image of all those soldiers who had preceded me—men who create a lineage spanning generations— wiping the rain from their eyes and putting the needs of others before their own. The beauty of the human spirit is glimpsed in the willingness of these individuals to be in this situation at all. At another level, this old saying is also a reminder to young recruits not to assign difficulty undue importance. By forewarning us that it is always 3 A.M., that we will always be peering through rain, in the dark, at the edges of two quickly disintegrating maps, our elders are also confirming that it is in our nature to be able to rise to such challenges.

Most of us have high hopes concerning our practice of yoga and our ability to live our yoga. We entertain lofty visions of newfound equanimity, of a harmonious balance between our inner lives and our outer reality. Unfortunately, most of us spend our days in something short of this vision. Raising children, loving partners, sitting in traffic, waiting anxiously for botched election returns, spilling orange juice on the good suit, or taking an aging parent out to dinner, we must constantly adjust our ideal in order to accommodate real life. We often find that it is 3 A.M., raining, and we are at the intersection of two maps, when the world most needs us to live our yoga. But we can do it. And we will do it beautifully.

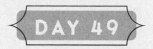

DAY 49

We are to think of ourselves as immortals, dwelling in the light, encompassed and sustained by spiritual powers. The steady effort to hold this thought will awaken dormant and unrealized powers, which will unveil to us the nearness of the eternal.

Charles Johnston

There are two lessons in this beautiful statement about yoga. The first concerns our true nature, "dwelling in the light, encompassed and sustained by spiritual powers." Either we believe in our innate goodness and beauty or we do not; it is up to each of us to decide. We may spend our entire lives believing a lie about our true nature, or we may put our trust in our own grace. Either way, most of us have to choose what we believe about ourselves each day, each hour, each moment of our lives. The Yoga Sutras suggest that we stand in our divinity, that we consciously experience ourselves as miraculous.

In the second sentence, Charles Johnston returns us to one of the central truths of the Yoga Sutras: that energy is like a muscle; it grows when we use it. We grow in our capacity to do the right thing each time we do the right thing. Steady effort to hold this thought will awaken dormant and unrealized powers within us, which will bring us closer to that which we seek. So our divinity is affirmed, and the manner in which we can make manifest this divinity is outlined. We believe and act accordingly, and as we do, this belief grows in our life. We believe in compassion, live compassion, and compassion grows in our lives. We believe in love, live lovingly, and love grows in our lives. We stand in our light, live our light, and the light grows within us. We need only make a beginning, and that beginning will foster within us the power to move forward.

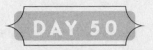

DAY 50

Where there is firm conquest over covetousness, they who have conquered it wake up to the how and why of life.

Yoga Sutras

The final *yama* is *aparigraha,* or nonpossessiveness and nonhoarding. As befits the end point of such a journey, *aparigraha* is about letting go. The Yoga Sutras advise us not to waste any energy holding on to that which is not really ours in the first place. As I write this, in the United States in the twenty-first century, it's hard not to sound like a Northeastern liberal know-it-all. The fact that we spend more on defense than on education begs the question "What are we defending and why are we defending it?" Wrapped up in this ongoing political debate is the wisdom and the message of *aparigraha.* The energy we expend defending unhealthy attachments could be spent making the world a better place.

Aparigraha applies to our own thinking as well. Attachment to our thoughts is as wasteful as our attachment to political ideology, to relationships, or to our piles of stuff. I have agonized over my own glacial progress around gender inequities. I was born on the cusp of the women's movement and grew up watching the roles of men and women change, transmute, become blurred, become indecipherable. Despite my love of women and my lifelong support for the underdog, I continue to struggle with my concept of life as a zero-sum game, my automatic assumption that if you win, I lose. I read about women now outnumbering men in law schools, and I shudder with images of my own future powerlessness—despite the fact that I have no desire whatsoever to go to law school. This irrational fear of "women's lib"—and it was in the air at the time of my birth—has to some extent poisoned my soul. It is time to let go, to clean house both inside and out. *Aparigraha* is also about letting go of our most cherished pain-producing beliefs. It is about the end of all attachment: letting go of our fears, letting go of our desires, becoming free.

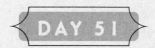

DAY 51

The mark of a moderate woman is freedom from her own ideas.

Lao-Tzu

Aparigraha advises us to travel light while on the spiritual path. We must let go of the old to make room for the new; we must grieve our dead and then let go in order to love the living. Much of the work we do with *aparigraha* concerns the obvious. We can't use a closet if it is stuffed full of worn-out clothing. We don't like the new office staff because we have not said good-bye to the old staff. As difficult as these passings are, they have the advantage of being directly in front of us. All that is required is yet another level of surrender, a leap of faith.

More difficult is the aspect of *aparigraha* that concerns worn-out beliefs. Many of the basic assumptions that guide our daily choices are unconscious, unseen. We have assimilated Uncle Ted's advice on tire purchases, Aunt Liv's guidance concerning the color red, the sixth-grade bully's contempt for the

Red Sox, an entire lifetime of half-heard conversations and misinterpreted advice—and it all figures somehow into our daily decision making.

My mother told me over and over again, "We come from a house of manners." In fact, this was not true, but I hear her words in my mind to this day. The point is, we have all been programmed, sometimes intentionally, sometimes unintentionally, to an extent that most of us are only vaguely aware of. Of equal power are our own beliefs, carried over from previous periods of our lives, previous life situations. Collectively, these old thoughts and ideas are an energy in our lives that rob us of the moment. *Aparigraha* invites us to walk away from yesterday's outdated beliefs. Just as we take boxes of our old clothing to the Salvation Army, we can begin shedding our old ideas. Yesterday's definition of a man or a woman, a race or a religion, a blessing or a curse no longer has any power over us. We can begin to trust our perceptions of the truth in the moment. There is a power in this process, an unfettering of the mind and the spirit. We can begin to wear our beliefs like a loose garment. We can experience the lightness that comes from freedom from our own ideas.

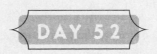

DAY 52

The spiritual life is always about letting go. It is never about holding on.

The Reverend Jesse Lee Peterson

Jesse is my meditation teacher. A modern-day saint whose ministry is in Los Angeles, Jesse uses meditation as the cornerstone of a set of practices that are effectively taking on the most difficult issues of our day. His students come from all walks of life, and those who have followed his teachings have been uniformly successful. When asked recently who today is following in the footsteps of her father, Martin Luther King Jr.'s youngest daughter singled Jesse out as her father's spiritual heir, the leader whose message captures the essence of King's teachings. One of Jesse's teachings captures the essence of *aparigraha* as well.

The first step on Jesse's road to wellness is forgiveness. The anger we hold on to, he says, owns us and poisons us. For years I had meditated, practiced yoga, prayed, and performed service, yet I could not be rid of my anger. Traffic, phone bills, my wife, my dog, my friends, and my enemies—all were quite capable of inspiring my irrational resentment. I could not understand why I had made so little progress with my anger, until Jesse spelled it out for me. As long as I was angry with anyone, I harbored anger, and I was therefore an angry person. Reflecting on this, I was quickly able to come up with a list of resentments that were many years old. I had written about these resentments, taken responsibility for them, talked of them in therapy, but I had never forgiven the individuals in question. Without the cleansing decision to forgive, I continued to be resentful, and I continued to be angry. Many of my resentments were *aparigraha* violations. I not only held onto these resentments but cherished them. I hoarded them. Yet I remained perplexed about the fact that anger lived in me.

Jesse told me, as he has told tens of thousands of others, that I would not be free in a spiritual sense until I did the work of forgiveness. I had to go back to each of those people I had harbored resentment toward, speak honestly about the particulars of our relationship, and formally forgive them. Only after I had let go of these old animosities would I be truly free. To the protests of "Yeah, but I am different" or "Yeah, but this situation is different" or "Yeah, but So-and-so is dead" or "Yeah, but So-and-so would never speak to me even if I tried," Jesse answers, "The spiritual life is always about letting go. It is never about holding on." Let go and be free.

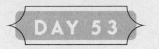

T H E   Y A M A S

Peace is the first condition, without which nothing else can be stable.

Sri Aurobindo

Yesterday's essay concerned the connection between forgiveness, letting go, and freedom. As I wrote it, I could almost hear the chorus of objections piping up across the country. So I decided to spend a little more time today on the concept of forgiveness. Yoga de-ages us. Our spines become supple, our muscles grow firm and youthful. We regain physical powers lost to us for many years, if we ever had them in the first place. Forgiveness does for the soul and for our relationships what the postures do for our bodies.

I recently spent time with a cherished old friend. Under Jesse's influence, I apologized for my wrongdoing in our relationship and forgave him for those occasions when he had wronged me. We have been friends for ten years, and over that time unsettled grievances had aged our relationship, blocking the intimacy that was once there. By doing the hard work of making amends and asking for and granting forgiveness, we were able to renew our friendship and make it fresh. We could be beginners again; our friendship was made young once more.

Yes, you may say, but what about the people I don't cherish? What about the horrible uncle who terrorized me as a child and couldn't care less? What about my parents, who violated me and deny it ever happened? What about the people whose racism or sexism denied me the innocence of my childhood? Why should I forgive those who do not seek forgiveness and do not deserve it?

Forgiveness can never be entirely self-serving. We do forgive others for our own spiritual growth, but the most important reason for forgiveness is

PART ONE

The Beginning

70

our belief in interconnectedness. Because we are all one, what we cannot forgive in others we cannot forgive in ourselves; what we withhold from others we withhold from ourselves. The judgments we pronounce upon others are ultimately being pronounced upon ourselves, because there is no you and no me, there is only we. Forgiveness, therefore, is an act of self-love, and by loving ourselves we love the whole of humanity. Ensnared in our own condemnation, we can find no peace. Forgiveness frees us from this predicament and lays the foundation upon which our spiritual life can be built.

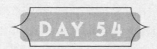

DAY 54

You're not a hoarder, you're a nonrelinquisher.

Eleanor Williams

On Tuesdays I spend an hour with my *pranayama* instructor, Eleanor Williams. An exceedingly wise and witty teacher from the Iyengar tradition, Eleanor has been a source of great support during the writing of this book. Our time together is spent in a large formal dining room, complete with a crystal chandelier, that she has converted into a studio. With the afternoon light spilling across the impeccable wood floor, Eleanor puts me through my paces. We usually begin our sessions with a little yoga chat. Last week I informed her that I was coming to the end of the *yamas* and had found the experience of writing about them to be life transforming. I mentioned *aparigraha* to her and described the condition of my rented storage space (very, very full). She smiled and said, "You're not a hoarder, you're a nonrelinquisher."

With these words I suddenly saw the work I still need to do on *aparigraha* in a new light. I've gone into great detail about the fact that, out of unreasoning fear, we hold on to concepts and objects that would be better shared or let go. Nevertheless, Eleanor held up a mirror for me, and in it I saw reflected my own deep-seated belief that once I have something, I had better hold on to it, whatever it is. This is not about coveting or hoarding or greed. It is just fear in another color—the fear that comes from want. It is the fear of those who have done without.

At first glance, *aparigraha* sounds like a problem of the shop-till-you-drop club. But upon further examination, I realized that my whole apartment is one big *aparigraha* violation. I am not a big spender, and I hardly ever shop. So how can this be? I don't want more, I just don't want to lose what I already have. I might miss that shirt I haven't worn in years. I might want to read that book again someday. That chipped bowl is still perfectly usable. It's not that I am a hoarder, I am a nonrelinquisher. I don't want to grieve the loss of anything. *Aparigraha* is an opportunity to learn how to say good-bye.

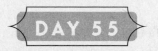

DAY 55

Fortunately, healthy people experience almost daily flashes of vision—the peak experience—which makes us aware that there is something badly wrong with our basic assumptions: they bring the flash of "absurd good news."

Colin Wilson

Aparigraha embodies the idea of good things to come. Once we realize that we can actually part with whatever it is we have been holding on to—the ten-year-old T-shirts with sentimental value, the receipts we never turned in, the clutter of our lives—we begin to understand that we are clearing a space for something better. The past is dead, and we are making room for the living. I like to think of this kind of housecleaning as analogous to the preparations an expectant couple make for their baby, transforming the guest room into a nursery. There is the same sense of potent expectancy as we embrace *aparigraha* and set out to audaciously clean house.

One of the ways I'm learning to let go is with bills. In the last few years I've stopped paying the minimum and begun paying my bills in full. Somewhere along the way, I came to understand that the money I gave to my creditors wasn't really mine in the first place, and that paying the minimum each month was just a way to prolong an unsatisfactory relationship. Years of yoga have finally brought me to the obvious conclusion that the only way I can end my indebtedness is by paying off my debts. All of them. The *yamas* are simply a means to reclaim our own energy. The money I owe MasterCard may not be mine, but the energy tied up in the state of indebtedness is. Oftentimes when we believe that we've been holding on to something we need, we find that the reverse is actually true. The real loss is the emptiness, the soul sickness, that we feel around any form of fear disguised as greed or hoarding. The symbols of our fear block us from the light of our own spirit. As we step away from these symbols, these phantoms, a wind catches our sails. Lighter, freer, we look up and glimpse the far shore, and suddenly we are filled with the joy of "absurd good news."

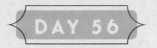

When you can fall for chains of silver you can
fall for chains of gold.

Dire Straits

We are a fortunate generation in a fortunate country, and most of us have been able to have our material wants gratified many times over. We have also experienced the emptiness behind "more," behind the idea that our insides can be made right by something or someone outside ourselves. Yet there remains a tension. We continue to choose the bondage of materialism because we cannot believe that we will ever be free.

Behind the impulse to find a solution outside ourselves is the pain of being lost. We often react in our day-to-day lives like people in pain. I was in a body cast for thirteen weeks when I was eleven. One night I had to go to the bathroom and no one in my family was awake to help me. Fading in and out of sleep, I dreamt I had a tank that I drove up to the house and fired, and that the cannon woke everybody up. Eventually my father came and all was well, but this piece of wishful dreaming has stayed with me. I believe that many of us in pain regularly fall into thinking and problem solving that are no more rational than my childhood dream. If I have a date for Saturday night, I will feel better about myself. If I were thin, I would have the life I have always wanted. A million dollars is not enough; I need to figure out how to earn more.

Of course, the pain of being lost is eased when we finally do find our way back home. This is the aim of yoga. When we seek answers outside ourselves, we go deeper into the wilderness, further from home. *Aparigraha* is about recognizing our fears and letting them go. We hold on to that which is not really ours in the first place because we are afraid. We hold on to outworn beliefs because we are afraid. We are willing to believe that something outside ourselves will make us whole because we are afraid. Being afraid does not make us right, it only makes us unhappy. *Aparigraha,* like all of the *yamas,* does not create our unhappiness, nor does it free us. We do that for ourselves. *Aparigraha* simply calls a chain a chain, whether it is made out of silver or made out of gold.

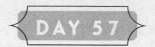

DAY 57

> Most of our energy goes into upholding our importance. If we were capable of losing some of that importance, two extraordinary things would happen to us. One, we would free our energy from trying to maintain the illusory idea of our grandeur; and two, we would provide ourselves with enough energy to catch a glimpse of the actual grandeur of the universe.
>
> Carlos Castaneda

Here is the essence of *aparigraha,* the *yama* that invites us to let go of the false self and all its symbols. As long as we are holding on to the thoughts and symbols of the false self, we are blocked from the sunlight of the spirit. In class, I say that if your hands are closed, they are not ready to receive a gift. Similarly, a closed fist blocks the flow of energy that yoga is intended to generate. When we arrive on our mats, we can begin our practice by combing our bodies, our minds, and our hearts, looking for the closed fist. *Aparigraha* is about taking the spiritual stance of an open hand. When we open our hands, when we open ourselves, we are ready to receive support from the universe.

On a practice level, *aparigraha* can free us from many an unpleasant burden. When I left the service, I embarked on a long sojourn into the realm of hand-to-mouth living. I delivered packages, waited tables, and worked as an EMT. It was a good time for me. I was learning about myself and God, but no one seemed to want to pay me while I was doing this. A couple of years into this process, I realized that my car, which had been perfectly affordable when I was in the army, was now eating up almost half my income. I was also well aware that my car represented the last vestige of the prestige I had enjoyed as a military officer. It assured me that my status as a waiter was temporary; soon I would get into my car and drive off to bigger and better things. Unfortunately, I had no such plans. The type of work I was attracted to paid even less than I was making as a waiter. In the meantime, I had to work much harder than my peers just to maintain the same standard of living. The time I spent working to support my car was time and energy that I could not spend supporting my spirit. Eventually, I sold my car and bought a bike. Soon after, I took a night off from work and rode out into a fragrant spring evening. As my tires glided silently over streets wet from a warm rain, I looked up through the trees and saw the stars come out as the clouds began to part. Alone, in silence, I caught a glimpse of the grandeur of the universe.

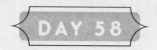

All that I want for you, my son, is to be satisfied. And be a simple kind of man, someone you can love and understand . . .

Lynyrd Skynyrd

Once we open ourselves to it, we find yoga everywhere. It is in the wind, it is in the grass and in the trees. The homecoming that is yoga is both the conflict and the resolution of the great myths, and the plot line of the TV sitcom. In the words of Jack Kornfield, "It is where we began and where we return."

This Lynyrd Skynyrd song was very meaningful to me in the fall of 1981, just over twenty short years ago. At the time, I was a teenager with a severe substance abuse problem, and I could not have told you why this song was so deeply stirring to me. All that I knew at the time was that my life was not simple, and the concept of a simple man who finds love was one I could get behind. Long before I was ready to do anything about it, the message of yoga was swirling around me. It came to me through athletics. It came to me in the form of caring advisers and friends. And it came to me in the form of an endless series of consequences.

On the mat I have learned not to live too fast. Troubles have come and they have passed. I found a woman and I found love. And I try never to forget that there is something up above. I've learned not to lust, and to believe that what I need is in my soul. I follow my heart and nothing else. I've become a simple man who I can love and understand. I am satisfied.

PART ONE

The Beginning

1

DAY 59

Do not take counsel of your fears.

General Barry McCaffrey

So we have come to the end of the *yamas*. Nonviolence, honesty, nonstealing, moderation, nonhoarding. A lifetime of work, the foundation of a happy life—summed up in five words. These five words define the saint and inform the rest of us. Whenever I am disturbed by a person or a situation, I now go through this five-word checklist to discover the source of my disturbance. Invariably, the *yamas* lead me back into myself, back to some fear I am harboring. Living the *yamas* is at once an awesome challenge and a simple task. At their core is personal responsibility. We are faced over and over again with a choice: to take responsibility for our fear or to deny it. Over and over again, we are called upon to see that we can make our decisions from a place of fear or from a place of faith.

I still remember a speech I heard in 1987 as a young army officer. A handsome gray-haired Southern gentleman of an officer was addressing a group of us, all recently graduated from college. For most of us, being an officer in the U.S. Army was our first experience as adults. General McCaffrey was a compassionate man, and his aim was to help us through this difficult time of transition. He told us that we had all been fortunate; we were gifted young people, and so the world had beaten a path to our doors. Now we were embarking on a new journey, during which we would routinely be held responsible for situations that were out of our control. He advised us not to become embittered or to lose heart in the face of setbacks. "Do not take counsel of your fears," he said. I have not forgotten this man's advice. Over the years, I've found these words to be simple, applicable to any situation, and profound. This is the pathway to peace and the message of the *yamas*. In the pages of this book, we are leaving the *yamas* now, but the *yamas* will never leave us. As you live in the company of the guiding spirits that are the *yamas,* you do so held in my prayers and with my wish that you will not take counsel of your fears.

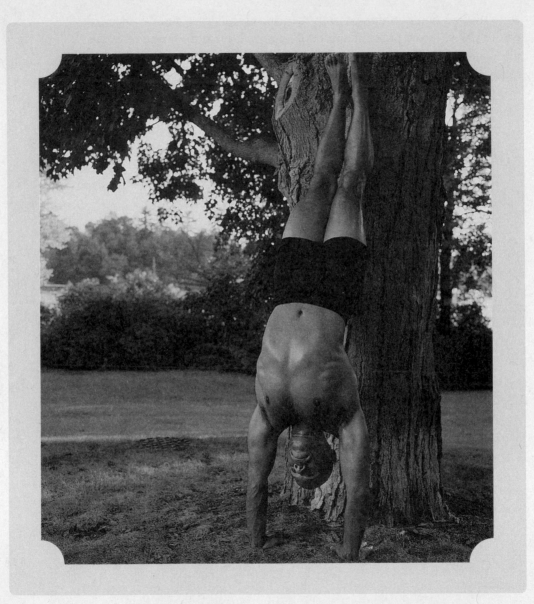

PART TWO

THE NIYAMAS

Sustaining Practices

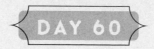

> We swing the sword not to learn to cut flesh, but to develop the will to adhere to our beliefs.
>
> Japanese sword master

The *yamas* are in many ways the hardest work on this path, for they confront us with the enormous challenge of rechanneling our spiritual energies. The *yamas* form the very bedrock of our existence. Before encountering the *yamas,* we are prey to the whims of our minds. Our minds tell us we are good, so we feel good; our minds tell us we are bad, so we feel bad. Our orientation is outward; we continuously compare ourselves to others, and most of the time we find ourselves lacking. We search outside ourselves for the validation we crave. And since we have no control over this validation, we can never truly be at peace or gain access to our true power in this life. The *yamas* change all of this. The energy we have poured into fruitless effort now becomes redirected into a process that gains us lasting peace and freedom. The *yamas* are the fundamental renunciation of a life based on fear. They are the change. The *niyamas* are the fundamental practices that sustain a life based on love. They sustain the change.

As is true of the *yamas,* the essence of the *niyamas* is found in every major religion. They have been passed down to us in this form by our spiritual brothers and sisters who have gone before us. These are the practices that have been found, over thousands of years, to support the individual who has chosen a spiritual path. Purity, contentment, zeal in practice, self-study, and devotion are habits that keep us from spiritual harm and sustain us in our faith as we live in this world. Like the swing of the sword master's blade, they sustain within us the will to adhere to our beliefs.

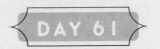

We have never stayed home long enough to experience the
truth about ourselves.

Erich Schiffmann

To properly understand the *niyamas,* or any of the practices of the yoga path, we must see them in terms of this observation by yoga teacher Erich Schiffmann. The second yoga sutra states, "Yoga is the cessation of movements in the consciousness." Yoga is a means for us to become still, to come home. The *niyamas* are an ancient set of practices, founded on the truths common to all of the great religions, that promote stillness in the practitioner. But what exactly is stillness? And what's so great about it? What if you were a race car driver? Wouldn't it make more sense to study movement instead?

The simplest way to think about stillness is to first consider the state of anxiety, or agitation. This condition is the opposite of equipoise. If you are anxious or tense, you are drawn out of your center, you are out of balance. When you feel calm and collected, however, you are in balance. Asana practice gives us an excellent firsthand experience of the difference between the two states. In one, we struggle ineffectively, distracted, learning nothing, moving a lot, accomplishing little. In the other, we are balanced, still; without moving, we accomplish everything. Perfectly balanced, motionless in a yoga posture, we are able to catch a glimpse of the intersection of energy, matter, and awareness. We transcend ordinary consciousness and connect to a deeper reality. In stillness, we are able to have direct knowledge of our souls, to grasp the underlying reality of existence. Having experienced that stillness on the mat, we step back into our everyday lives with increased coordination and grace. And if you are a race car driver, practicing stillness will certainly make you a better one.

The *niyamas* are practices that we can bring into our daily lives to foster stillness, to bring us ease of heart. Each aspect of my day lends itself to a different *niyama* because each moment of my day offers me the opportunity to choose between pain or peace. A typical day might go like this: In the morning, I practice cleanliness, zeal in practice, and devotion. At work, I practice self-study, zeal in practice (remember, we are always practicing), and contentment. I finish my day with devotion and I go to bed with contentment. I practice these observances out of a desire to avoid the chaos that comes of *not* practicing them, and out of a desire to know the truth about myself.

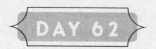

DAY 62

Cleanliness of the body and mind develops disinterest in
contact with others for self-gratification.

Yoga Sutras

The first *niyama* is *sauca,* or purity. Practicing *sauca,* we keep ourselves clean on the outside through ordinary means, and we keep ourselves clean on the inside through asana, *pranayama,* right eating practices, and right attitudes. I am not going to tell you what to eat, how often to bathe, which asana you should do when, or how to practice *pranayama.* But I do encourage you to weave these practices thoughtfully into your life. As far as the particulars go, follow the teachings of your guides and of your heart. I found an asana practice that works for me by being open to any teacher who was generous enough to teach me. I've developed a *pranayama* practice by seeking out someone who studied for many years under outstanding teachers. My personal hygiene is a work in progress, but its foundation was laid by the U.S. Army. As far as food goes, nothing could be more personal. *Sauca* is not about *what* we eat but about the cleanliness of our choices. When it comes to our thoughts, the entire practice of yoga is really concerned with this aspect of *sauca*. *Sauca*'s contribution is the practice of compassion. It is the observance of loving-kindness in thought.

Unlike the other *yamas* and *niyamas, sauca* receives two sutras of explanation. The work we do with *sauca* is primarily physical, but in both sutras the desired effect is in the mind. I think of *sauca* as the feng shui aspect of the Yoga Sutras, the moment where Patanjali acknowledges the effect of our environment—both mental and physical—on the state of our minds. As we practice yoga, we are to be aware of both aspects of *sauca*—the *sauca* we do on the mat and that which we do while off the mat. On the mat, begin to experience the asana and *pranayama* as purifying your body as well as strengthening it. Off the mat, cultivate consciousness and care around the choices you make concerning your mental and physical environment. Begin with your physical cleanliness, your grooming habits, the cleanliness of your clothes, and then work outward. How are your surroundings affecting you? Make your bed, clean the bathtub, and wash the dishes—then ask yourself the question again: How are my thoughts creating my emotional reality? Think of five things to be grateful for in this day, and then ask yourself this question again. Over time, as you apply the principle of *sauca* to your life, you will find that a peace settles over you. As you no longer turn to "contact with others for self-gratification," you will begin to experience the freedom and joy that is *sauca*.

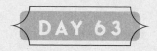

When the body is cleansed, the mind purified and the senses
controlled, joyful awareness, needed to realize the
inner self, also comes.

Yoga Sutras

The second sutra concerning *sauca* speaks to the energetic experience of
purifying and cleansing. We practice *sauca* and we become happy. Erich
Schiffmann has written that as we deepen our yoga practice, we become
happy for no apparent reason. To experience progress on this path *is* to
become happy for no apparent reason, as we fundamentally change the way
we move through our days. In fact, our lives change so radically that we forget why it was we were unhappy in the first place. Our newfound happiness
appears to be for no reason. In truth, however, we are happy because we
have applied the principles of yoga to our lives.

When I first began to understand the principles of yoga and to examine
my thoughts from this new perspective, I realized that I already had a fully
formed philosophy of life. Unfortunately, my philosophy was a hodge-
podge of overheard conversations, mistaken briefs, rantings of people in pain,
TV ads, media propaganda, and so on. Garbage in, garbage out. My life was
a reflection of all the thoughts I allowed to dominate my mind as I moved
through my days. The script was quite miserable. Here are a few highlights:
"I am defined by my gender, race, and accomplishments." "The highest
form of acknowledgment and approval is if you have sex with me." "There
will always be people whose lives are better than mine." "I am deeply
ashamed of who I have been and must conceal my real self from you." "You
will like me if I am impressive." Does any of it sound familiar?

If we are to find lasting happiness, we must not only clean up our rooms but clean up our thoughts as well. Fortunately, that is precisely what the practice of yoga is all about. To begin, we let go. We let go of our thoughts, our old scripts, our expectations, our darkness. The solution is not to fight but to let go. We let go of everything and hold on to nothing. Over and over again, on the mat and off, we let go. This letting go is a purification. We let go and it is like dropping a pebble into a pond, the ripples slowly growing to encompass our every waking moment. In our letting go we create an emptiness, a space that health and grace will move into. We begin to live with a joyful awareness.

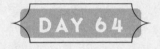

DAY 64

Hint: the cage is not locked.

Nova Knutson

Sauca is the moment on our path when we begin to take the maintenance of our physical condition seriously. My own beginnings were quite humble. I spent the last few years before my spiritual awakening routinely going for weeks without a shower, sleeping on the ground, smoking a pack of cigarettes a day, eating military rations that had been prepared years before, drinking as much alcohol as I could whenever I could, and wondering why I felt so bad most of the time. True, this was my job description, but it was also a job that I had chosen in the throes of spiritual bankruptcy.

Once I had emerged from that spiritual nadir and begun a spiritual practice, I started to look around. The people I admired seemed to be treating their bodies well. They appeared to have some principles about their food, their behavior, their beliefs and attitudes. They exercised, wore clean clothes, lived in clean apartments. There was a gentleness in all of this. I had a sense that these habits were an extension of the love these individuals felt toward themselves and others. I had exercised to win competitions, and I'd ironed my uniforms to pass military inspections, but I had never thought of these activities as a means of taking care of myself. *Sauca* confirms my observations of my early role models. Our body is the home of our spirit. It is the means by which we enact our beliefs. Therefore, the maintenance of the body is a spiritual duty, an act of love not only toward ourselves but toward all humanity.

Practicing *sauca,* we are also turning belief into action. We have embraced a path that is about freedom and love. As we care gently and lovingly for ourselves, we are deconstructing the blocks to love in our lives and freeing ourselves from the prison of outworn patterns of thought and action. And we need to start somewhere. Yoga says we should start where we are, on the physical plane, with our bodies and the acts of our bodies. Furthermore, we must begin to see our minds as organs of action, and our thoughts as acts. Each step we take on this path is a step into the unknown and a confirmation of our ability to live a better life. The people whose practice of *sauca* I watched and admired early on in my spiritual journey were actually doing it: they were enacting their spiritual beliefs in a tangible, everyday way. *Sauca* is an invitation to spread your wings a little bit, to experience your freedom, to take small steps with big consequences, to break free. Go ahead. Hint: the cage is not locked.

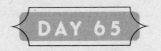

DAY 65

Move a muscle, change a feeling.

Anonymous

The old adage "Move a muscle, change a feeling" accurately describes the gist of yogic theory. We begin with the external and work inward. Many of us grew up in homes where *sauca* was practiced as a matter of course. The floors were clean, the beds made, and there was a sense of safety and peace in the orderliness of it all. But many others of us grew up in chaos. I grew up in a home that was physically orderly but emotionally chaotic. I rebelled against this, and sought emotional order amidst physical chaos. My resentments have not been a great plan for living.

Wherever you find yourself on the *sauca* continuum, *sauca* remains two things. First, it is a leap of faith, because we are often too tired, too sad, or too angry to believe that anything will really make a difference. And second, it is an everyday practice, because yesterday's *sauca* serves only as a reminder of today's potential.

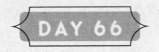

DAY 66

As a result of contentment, one gains supreme happiness.

Yoga Sutras

The second *niyama* is *santosa,* or contentment. This is the choice to end our war with reality. In the world in which I grew up, there were winners and there were losers, and you were either one or the other. Winning was great and losing sucked. My internal reality was dictated by external events, and I never questioned it. In a happy ending, the bad guy gets taken out and the good guy gets the girl, or something like that. This assumption was based on my belief that there were unhappy endings. Despite the endless emotional ups and downs, and the years of anxiety this belief system produced, it was only much later, after significant good fortune, that I even began to question the emotional roller-coaster I called daily life.

At twenty-six, I lost completely at the game of substance abuse. Not only was I no longer able to pull it off, I was remanded to treatment, where I had to turn in my "party guy" label and don the dubious label of "addict." Due to the enormous pain I was in, I surrendered. While those around me in treatment fought last-ditch battles, a few others and I just threw in the towel. As the dust settled and the days passed, I came to see that the very depth of my surrender had provided me with the spiritual strength to move on. While those around me who refused to admit defeat were still stuck in a seemingly perpetual cycle of denial and pain, my life was already changing. I was in recovery—and suddenly life felt like a whole new ball game. Maybe losing wasn't so bad. Up until that point, I had seen the struggle for control as the only game in town. In fact, I had never viewed it as a struggle; I thought it was just life. Having surrendered all in order to survive, I now began to see an alternative way of moving through the world.

Santosa is just that—an alternative way to move through the world. It is a shift of focus. Instead of seeking contentment from the outside in, we find contentment from the inside out. The paradigm shift comes when we view all events as opportunities to grow, to encounter our own magnificence. When we view things in this light, there are no good events or bad events, only moments in which to shine.

DAY 67

> We can easily practice *santosa* in the beautiful moments and
> joyous experiences of our lives. But Patanjali asks us to be
> equally willing to embrace the difficult moments.
>
> Judith Lasater

Personally, I think that practicing contentment in the beautiful moments is not a bad place to start. I've spent countless high points in my life fretting over this aspect or that aspect of the moment: Will it last? Is it real? Am I worthy? Blah, blah, blah. It has been an ongoing struggle for me to be content in the beautiful moments, to be still in success. I am much better at setbacks. My childhood was a study in setbacks. I endured racism, abuse, and addiction. Paradoxically, my struggles taught me that God is with me, that I can trust the universe, and that tomorrow will in fact be another day. Although I have far less experience with things *not* falling apart, as I write these words, my life is all that I ever hoped it would be. And yet, my challenge now is to practice *santosa*. My yoga practice right now, all of it—the postures, the prayers, the *pranayama,* the meditation, and the work off the mat—is devoted to being still while things are going well. My practice is devoted to things being enough.

Santosa is the practice of being still with faith, with an open heart and an open mind. We have an opportunity to do this in the postures that we like and the postures that we don't like. Watch your reaction as you move from posture to posture. Where does your mind go when things are going well? Where does your mind go when things are hard? Can the moment be enough?

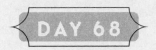

DAY 68

> Everyone is already the living Buddha, complete, whole, perfect
> as you are. All this action and effort to become special is just
> making you very unspecial and creating a tremendous amount of
> pain and suffering.
>
> Zen master Dennis Genpo Merzel

In a world in which we are not enough, the practice of contentment appears unwarranted. Before we can begin to make *santosa* a regular aspect of our experience, we must first confront the *avidya,* or spiritual ignorance, behind our striving and dissatisfaction. Any effort that begins with the belief "I am an imperfect person acting in an imperfect universe" will be in opposition to the aims of yoga. The practice of contentment begins with an awareness of how we evaluate ourselves and our surroundings.

In the military I was taught the art of land navigation with a map and a compass, and over the years, as I grew competent at navigation, I developed habits that kept me from getting lost. The most important habit was the precise establishment of the start point. The use of a map involves rudimentary geometry, and all of the calculations you make are based on your original estimation of where you began. If your start point is off, none of your subsequent calculations will bear any connection to reality. Happiness is like that. The work we do to find happiness flows from the manner in which we have defined ourselves. To begin, simply shift focus. When you experience conflict or discontent, stop and get a sense of your start point. What are the original calculations that have brought you to this point? Are you striving to be special when you already are?

DAY 69

Remember, you are God's son in whom he is well pleased.

A Course in Miracles

How many of us believe this? From what I've learned about myself, and from those people who have shared honestly with me, most of us feel as though we are God's errant child, in whom she is greatly disappointed. We may talk the talk and even walk the walk of enlightenment, but in our hearts nothing really changes. We identify ourselves with our darkness, and nothing we do seems to change the status quo. We pray for ten years to become more tolerant, yet our minds still seem to be on autopilot. When the lady in front of us has fifteen items in the express lane at the whole-foods store—where we've gone to tread lightly on Mother Earth—she is no longer our sister but a deeply flawed being.

These feelings are at the heart of the work we do with *santosa*. We cannot practice contentment and continue to identify with our darkness. How often have you gone to yoga class with the intention of having a good practice, only to find yourself mired in distraction or judgment? Is it possible that distraction and judgment are not who you are? Is it possible that judgment or distraction are like the rain, and you are like the earth? The rain comes and goes, but the earth remains. To begin to feel *santosa,* learn to love the earth. You will soon experience yourself as the *jivatman,* or living spirit, in whom the universe is well pleased.

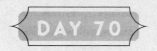

Already I could feel my being turned. Instinct and intellect
balanced equally. As in a wheel whose motion jars nothing.
By the Love that moves the Sun and the other stars.

Dante

There is an inner light that comes into the faces of those who have begun to walk the path. Initially, we are filled with self-conscious fear. Our postures are all about trying to get it right. We are practicing yoga with the same suppressed hopelessness with which we experience a life that doesn't quite work. Then, one bright morning or some dark evening, the energy begins to move. We wake from our spiritual winter. Oftentimes we are the last to see the difference. Those around us are captivated by the new sparkle in our eyes, a radiance that seems to shine from within, the bloom of health. Eventually we get it. Slowly we awaken to these barely perceptible changes, the outer manifestations of the profound shift that is taking place in our lives.

I experienced such a moment of clarity the spring after I returned home from the army. I had spent my last couple of years in college aware that I was preparing to enter a situation from which there was no guarantee of return. I had chosen to be an infantry officer in the U.S. Army under Ronald Reagan, and it was clear that we were gearing up for war. As a young infantry officer, I knew that if we did go to war, I would very likely meet my death. While my civilian peers prepared for their lives after college, I privately prepared for death. I had no regrets. All I had ever wanted to be was a warrior, and now I was either going to live—or to die as I wanted to. My training in the army only served to loosen my grip on life. I no longer harbored any illusions about the hazards of my profession. I did not experience my fatalism as a negative; in fact, I saw my role in our society as an honor.

Then one spring morning, just months after coming home from my stint overseas, I found myself jogging through the woods of Concord, Massachusetts. I still had not been able to fully grasp the fact of my survival. The country *had* gone to war. My fellow soldiers had killed thousands of Iraqi draftees; I had watched my own countrymen die in service. And yet I had been spared. There was no blood on my hands and I was alive.

As I ran that morning, something deep inside me cracked open. Suddenly, remarkably, I really felt the spring warmth, the dust of the road, the smell of the pine trees. I could feel how good it was to be home. This, I realized, was grace: to run to the rhythm of my breath; to feel the possibility of a human life, my life; to experience God's love on a spring morning. I was alive, and I could feel myself being turned by "the Love that moves the Sun."

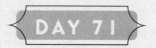

DAY 71

Do you want to improve the world? I don't think it can be done.
The world is sacred. It can't be improved.

Lao-Tzu

I have heard it said that words are inadequate to describe reality. At best, they are like pointing a finger at the moon in an attempt to describe the moon. Twenty-five hundred years ago, in the *Tao Te Ching,* Lao-Tzu pointed a finger to the essence of *santosa.* Contentment is not complacency, it is reverence. Yoga asks us to dip below the surface of the imperfect world created by our imaginations and connect to the divinity that underlies our existence. J. Krishnamurti wrote, "Have you ever sat very silently, not with your attention fixed on anything, not making an effort to concentrate, but with the mind very quiet, really still? . . . If you can listen in this way, listen with ease, without strain, you will find an extraordinary change taking place within you, a change which comes without your volition, without your asking; and in that change there is great beauty and depth of insight."

Come into any posture—warrior two will do—rest your eyes at one point, and just breathe into every cell in your body. Listen with every cell in your body. Experience the soles of your feet and the palms of your hands, the length of your spine, the sensation of air against your skin. Allow the posture to bring you deeply into the moment and you will experience contentment—not as resignation but as the vibrant experience of all living beings, as the song that is sung by a world that is sacred.

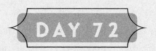

DAY 72

Behold, what I have seen to be good and to be fitting is to eat
and drink and find enjoyment in all the toil with which one toils
under the sun the few days of his life which God has given him.

Ecclesiastes 5:18

Leave it to the Old Testament to keep it real. Contentment is an everyday practice, and most of the time we will be applying it to our everyday responsibilities, our everyday toil. I am writing this morning at a bed-and-breakfast that allows my wife and me to bring our dog. The owner, Emily, breezes in to change our linen. The garden outside is glorious, and the accommodations inside are perfect, in a rough-and-ready New England way. Emily sees to all this with the ease and joy all happy people bring to their daily lives. There is a surrendering to the moment, certainly, but a respect as well. What else is there, after all, than the stuff of our daily lives? What could be more important than the manner in which we experience this very moment?

Marianne Williamson wrote that "the spiritual journey is the relinquishment—or unlearning—of fear, and the acceptance of love back into our hearts." Many of us have learned fear, and this has confused us. Many of us have experienced circumstances that were not OK, events that were not "all good." We have become afraid of suffering a repeat performance of these events or circumstances. In fact, most of us *will* lose someone we love again, or become ill for no reason, or lose a job, a child, a spouse. To contend with the fear our potential losses inspire, we tend to retreat into our imaginations. In her mid-seventies, Emily has endured it all—death, loss, war, and disease. We all do. They did back when Ecclesiastes was written. Our fear places conditions on our experience, but our love must still be unconditional and unconstrained. We must have the courage to embrace the days of our lives with faith and love. We can make peace with the past and with the future, as Emily has. And so we will find enjoyment in our toils under the sun.

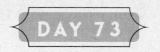

DAY 73

Lack of true knowledge is the source of all pains and sorrows.

Yoga Sutras

As we apply the principles of yoga, a profound understanding begins to resonate in our lives. We come to understand that the anxiety we feel, the suffering we experience, comes from *not* practicing yoga in the true sense of the word. Even the most tentative attempt at living our yoga produces immediate positive results. Bit by bit, we realize that we have been acting on misinformation and that all our strategies to end or lessen our suffering have actually intensified the pain.

Who among us has not lied to avoid suffering, only to have the lie increase her suffering tenfold? Who among us has not eaten a pint of Ben and Jerry's in the hope of feeling better for a moment, only to spend hours in regret? Who among us has not spent months or years believing that when this or that finally happens, we'll be content, only to find that the contentment we seek is somehow beyond our grasp? There is no end to these predicaments—until we adopt a new plan, a new paradigm, a new way of thinking. Yoga offers us a new plan. In truth, it is a very old plan, and it encompasses the only plan that has ever worked. You don't need to embrace the whole plan to gain from it, nor do you have to believe in every aspect of the plan for it to work. But if lack of true knowledge is the problem, then openness to new information must lead to the solution. All you need is the willingness to make a beginning, to turn yoga from theory into action.

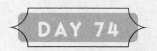

DAY 74

> Within us is a secret longing to remember the light, to step
> out of time in this dancing world. It's where we began
> and where we return.
>
> Jack Kornfield

This secret longing is the *why:* Why so much courage, why so much willingness, why so much pain, why so much joy, why so much life. Why we come back to our mats day after day. Why we remember who we are, and begin again, time after time, to come home to our true nature. Why we practice yoga.

We do it because we were born to. Just as a mother has no choice but to give birth to her child, we have no choice but to give birth to ourselves. This secret longing for the truth is where we began and where we return. Each step toward the light brings that much more peace to our hearts.

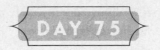

DAY 75

Self-discipline burns away impurities and kindles the sparks of divinity.

Yoga Sutras

The next *niyama* is *tapas,* or burning zeal in practice. This is right up our alley! Burning zeal in practice! A silent cheer rises up from the graves of our Puritan forefathers. "Now we are getting somewhere," you may think; "I knew there must be a way for me to fail to measure up. A chance to be able to cast my eye on my neighbor and just know that *they* are doing it right and I'm not, an opportunity to compete, a way to get ahead, a way to feel alternately inferior and superior, a way to screw this up."

All of this is true if *tapas* is not based in love for all beings, if our aim is not the end of suffering. *Tapas* is simply an enthusiasm for health. All of us have it; it is in our nature. The genius of yoga is that it encourages us to cultivate this enthusiasm. Rather than cloak our childlike wonder in cynicism, we are encouraged to develop an appetite for life.

In my own life there are three pillars that define my *tapas:* gratitude, a sense of wonder, and respect. The cornerstone of all of my spiritual work, and the prime mover in my *tapas,* is gratitude—a bone-deep gratitude for having been given a second chance at life, and for all of the magic that has happened since. The next aspect of my *tapas* is a sense of wonder. I am sure that I want to find out what happens next. I *believe* in the power of my practice, and I am eager to find out where this all leads. Finally, I am still impressed by the power of darkness. I have seen so many good people go under. I do not feel above the logic of karma, and therefore feel a prudent respect for the need to do the work.

When it comes to zeal in practice, begin by getting a sense of your underpinnings. At what level are you motivated? What fosters your zeal? What fosters your apathy? How will you kindle the sparks of divinity in your life?

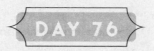

DAY 76

"Now," he thought, "that all these transitory things have slipped away from me again, I stand once more beneath the sun, as I once stood as a small child. Nothing is mine, I know nothing, I possess nothing, I have learned nothing . . ." He had to smile again. Yes, his destiny was strange! He was going backwards, and now he stood empty and naked and ignorant in the world. But he did not grieve about it; no, he even felt a great desire to laugh, to laugh at himself, to laugh at this strange, foolish world.

Hermann Hesse

Whenever I think of *tapas* burning away my impurities, I imagine it as the yogic equivalent of being in the fat-burning zone of exercise. I envision *tapas* burning off some of the toxins I consumed with my Chinese takeout last night. This is in fact the case. There is an aspect of our yoga practice that is simply about staying healthy. But a far more profound aspect of *tapas* is described above in the lines from *Siddhartha*.

The spiritual energy released by our practice strips away all that is false, the way a wind blows sand from the surface of a mirror. Most of us begin a spiritual practice having known only our false selves. And so, as those layers begin to fall away, it actually feels as if we are going backward at first, instead of forward; our practice strips away the edifice we built to our false self. Suddenly our whole way of knowing, of doing, of being comes into question. Our certainties fall away, along with the persona that we've long presented to the world. Many of us find that we have built our houses on sand, that the lives we've created cannot stand up to the heat of our practice. We may lose a job, relationships, the old playmates and playthings. We stand once more as a child in the world, open and empty. This, too, is *tapas*.

In my own life, I felt just as Siddhartha did—amazed at all I had lost, and at the same time just as amazed that I no longer valued what I had lost: my old self, the old world, the old friends . . . When two people who have experienced this aspect of *tapas* discuss it, it is invariably an occasion for much laughter—the laughter of relief at no longer needing to be our false self, and the laughter of joy at such good fortune.

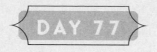

Explore daily the will of God.

C. G. Jung

Tapas is the spirit of inquiry; it is about having the heart of an explorer. It is the willingness to work hard in practice, the desire to know oneself, the will to be honest. But all of these virtues are predicated on a genuine desire for spiritual health. This desire will give us consistency. We will have good days and bad days, days when the spirit is willing but the flesh is weak, and days when the opposite is the case. Years of consistent practice are not built on rigid self-discipline; they are built on the desire to know more.

I recently attended a talk given by an uneducated man who had spent twenty years in prison for murder. In prison he had been extremely violent, and now that he is out, he is living on disability, in part owing to injuries incurred while in jail. About seven years ago, he had a spiritual awakening. While the particulars of his story are unique, its theme is universal. As a young man, his circumstances prepared him for a specific role in society. He embraced it, and for a while it worked for him. But his spiritual awakening occasioned a complete reevaluation of all his basic assumptions about life. In the years since, he has sought the guidance of a higher power and developed a new set of priorities. In his old life, things were predictable; in his new life, each day is an adventure. He ended his talk by saying that he sleeps well at night now, and that upon waking he feels guided through his days by a loving force. This man did not seek out *tapas*. *Tapas,* for him, is a natural reaction to the events of his life. He wakes each day with a lively desire to explore the will of God.

DAY 78

We have to keep in mind that we are learners, not judges.

Father Laurence

I spent a number of years working with adolescents who had grown up in chaotic circumstances. Having lived around adults who had very little control over their own behavior, these children had grown up with little sense of limits, boundaries, or consequences. A typical conversation between us might go like this: I would say, "Tommy, you cannot go out into the community with us today because you sprayed the executive director of the program with a garden hose while you were skipping class." Tommy would then swear and shout and tell me that the director was not a good person. I would spend ten minutes or so with Tommy, letting him know that while I was going to enforce the rules of the program, and see to it that he reaped the consequences of his actions, he had not lost my respect or affection.

Once Tommy understood that he had not lost his standing in our relationship, he would begin to find the confidence to try new behaviors. His old way would have been to blow up, reject the situation, and learn nothing. Held by our relationship, though, he was eventually able to try something new, listen to feedback from his peers, apologize, and begin to learn from his mistakes.

For many of us, our yoga teacher fulfills the role of steadfast advocate as we take risks and try new behaviors on the mat. In time, however, we must begin to be able to do this for ourselves. We must learn to trust that if we fall out of a balancing posture, rest during a vigorous class, or take a day off when we are tired, we will not lose our own respect or affection. Many of us expect more of ourselves than we would ever ask of anyone else. We simply cannot live up to our potential unless we are willing to live boldly and take adaptive risks. But if we are to continue to learn and grow, we must also know that at the end of the day there will be a home to return to, where we will be loved for our hearts as well as our deeds. We must be steadfast in our love and respect for ourselves, both when we soar and when we stumble.

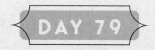

DAY 79

> How much of the world had I missed while living in my head? If each cell in our bodies is an outpost of our brains, what might I have learned? I'll never know who that adventurous little girl might have become. But at least I know that she's still there— waiting to enter the present.
>
> Gloria Steinem

It's hard to believe Gloria Steinem is not talking about yoga in this passage from her book *Moving Beyond Words.* Nevertheless, she articulates the essence of *tapas,* the yearning to know more, the desire to integrate lost selves, the passion to live fully. All of us are set on a trajectory by the circumstances of our birth, gender, class, family, and life experiences. The sum total of all these forces in our lives, and the choices we make concerning those forces, is our karma. Most of us simply enact our karma. Privilege begets privilege, disadvantage begets disadvantage. Recently I read about a study of human resiliency in which it was determined that the ability of individuals to overcome trauma was directly connected to their appearance. The primary indicator for success was good looks. To me, this indicates the extent to which most of us allow externals to define us. Karma is the momentum of all the external forces in our lives, including the consequences of choices we have made in the past. *Tapas* is the generation of internal momentum to counter-act the momentum of karma.

The spiritual journey can be likened to waking up one day to find one-self mindlessly floating down a river. The first step is to acknowledge that we are in a river. The second step is to understand that we have a choice about it. Many of us then try to swim upstream, but eventually we arrive at the third step: we get out of the river. If karma is the river, then *tapas* is the will to get out of the river. Earlier in her essay, Gloria Steinem writes about how her family, her gender, her culture, and the choices she made to con-tend with these influences had denied her the full use of her body. She goes on to describe her awakening and the forming of her desire to live more fully. The early stages of such a journey, during which we acknowledge and reclaim our lost selves, are quite painful. Grieving the harm we have done to ourselves is part of the process. Later, we must hold to the vision of a new life in the face of adversity. In both legs of the journey, *tapas* is the energy that sees us through. *Tapas* is the will both to look at what we have lost and to see what we can reclaim.

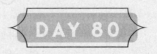

DAY 80

Desire, ask, believe, receive.

Stella Terrill Mann

Lao-Tzu wrote, "True words seem paradoxical." At the heart of *tapas* is desire, and at the heart of yoga is desirelessness. Both statements are true. Yoga defines desire as one of the basic problems in our lives. The desire to *have*—wanting—comes from a place of lack. We believe that we are imper-fect and that we need to fix ourselves. This is desire, and it only takes us deeper into our darkness. *Tapas,* or burning zeal in practice, is the will to attain spiritual health and to apply spiritual principles to our lives. These definitions of *tapas* appear to imply that our present situation is unsatisfactory and that right action will correct this. Stella Terrill Mann captures the real movement of *tapas,* from its inspiration in our hearts, to its formulation into action, through its maintenance, and finally to its fruition. *Tapas* begins in our hearts with a desire to be whole, to realize our potential, to come home. It is the manifestation of desire.

Tapas becomes yoga when it is enacted without attachment to results. For years I trained in a hot room under expert instruction. I was dedicated, and over time I developed the capacity of my body to a high degree. I overcame many internal obstacles in order to do this. This was wrestling, however, and in the end it was all about winning and losing. By making external events my priority, I remained defined by them, defined by my karma. Later, I once again spent years in a hot room under expert instruction. Over time, and with dedication, I developed the capacity of my body to a high degree. I overcame many internal obstacles in order to do this. This was yoga, and this time there were no winners and no losers. This journey became inwardly focused. I learned to practice without attachment to results. De-emphasizing the external, I have become progressively free from external influences, free from my karma. My work on that mat has become yoga.

In the first teaching of the Buddha—the teachings on the four
noble truths—he talked about suffering.

Pema Chodron

The Buddha began with suffering. A few years ago, it occurred to me that
the incomprehensible selfishness of certain men in power over the millennia can be explained by their assumption that an end to suffering could be
found outside themselves—and that with enough security, money, power,
or fame, an individual could escape suffering. I realized that *tapas* exists
whether we channel it into spiritual practice or not, for *tapas* is, essentially,
the drive to end suffering. *Tapas* is simply an energy, and it can work either
for us or against us. In the ascendance of a Stalin or a Saddam Hussein or
an Osama bin Laden, there is evidence of tremendous drive, a burning zeal
to live, to rule, to win. In the vast fortunes of the superrich in this country
there is evidence of a tremendous desire to surpass the limitations of life as
it has been lived. Our suffering begets the will to end suffering. The will to
end suffering becomes the *tapas* of yoga when it is grounded in personal
responsibility.

The *tapas* of a Stalin, or an abusive spouse, or the head of a tobacco
company is based on the belief that our suffering is caused by external
events. The *tapas* of yoga is based on the idea that our suffering is caused by
our *reaction* to external events. Viewed in this light, our suffering becomes
our teacher. The ever-present demon becomes the ever-present teacher.
Nonviolence becomes possible, truthfulness becomes possible, nonstealing
becomes possible, moderation becomes possible, nonhoarding becomes possible. The *yamas* are a natural outgrowth of yoga's interpretation of the cause
of our suffering. According to the yogic philosophy of the eight-limb path,

we always have everything we need. When we fail to believe this, we suffer. We are here to create spiritual health—and we each have our own personal trainer, in the form of our suffering. The greatest teacher who ever lived is our constant companion. The Buddha began with suffering because our understanding of our suffering defines the nature of our solution.

DAY 82

What is it that makes it so hard sometimes to determine whither we will walk? I believe that there is a subtle magnetism in Nature, which, if we unconsciously yield to it, will direct us aright.

Henry David Thoreau

In the early stages of my spiritual trek, I doggedly adhered to practice guidelines devised by individuals with far more experience than I had. I applied the findings of others to my own life with burning zeal. One mentor of mine worked on an ambulance while he took his premed courses, then went to medical school, so that is what I did. I went to school, became an EMT, worked on an ambulance, and took premed courses. After a year of full-time night work on an ambulance in Boston, I concluded that while the health care field was great for my friend, it definitely wasn't for me. This marked both the high-water mark of my rigid adherence to other people's visions and the moment when I began to find my own way.

Each one of us embarks on his or her yoga practice as a beginner, surrounded by more experienced practitioners. If we are earnest about our practice, if we have burning zeal, we will listen respectfully to those who have gone before us. Some of the advice we get will be life changing, some will be downright odd. We must learn to trust our own judgment on spiritual matters. But when we are just starting out, we must also be willing to trust the judgment of others, and to learn from them. Over time, our own wisdom awakens. When to practice, how to practice, what to practice—eventually the answers to all these questions will come to us from within. Each moment we live from the inside out strengthens our ability to do so in the future. Just as, at first, we must learn to yield to the wisdom of others, eventually we must learn to yield to the wisdom from within. As we do so, we see that it directs us aright.

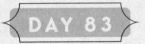

DAY 83

We will discover the nature of our particular genius when we stop trying to conform to our own or to other people's models, learn to be ourselves, and allow our natural channel to open.

Shakti Gawain

I recently went to see *Pollock,* a somber film about painter Jackson Pollock. For much of the film the audience is held captive to Pollock's addiction; his alcoholism is portrayed without sentiment or gloss. But in the midst of this gloom, there is a twenty-minute segment that is breathtaking. It is the moment when Pollock and his wife, who is also an artist, create a space for their art. They leave New York, get a house in the country, and construct a work space for painting. There is an excitement in these sequences as we realize that success is inevitable. Pollock and his wife seem to know it too—they come alive here, fully into their own powers. Suddenly their actions are deliberate and intentional, and there is a sense of inevitability, a knowing that such commitment will always bear fruit. And so, for a brief moment, the audience is able to go along for the ride, as two people say yes to their dharma. It is beautiful to watch.

As I was walking away from the movie, and in the days that followed, I reflected on the place I have assigned my own art in my life. Were someone to see my life on the big screen, would the boldness with which I have embraced my dharma be inspiring? What steps am I not taking, and why? Yoga tells us the time is now. We already have everything we need to be magnificent; it is simply a matter of allowing ourselves to be who we are. Suffering comes from our own resistance to being who we are. And so I am brought back to the questions of how and why I am choosing to suffer. Having felt the joy of doing what I was meant to do, and having witnessed that joy in others as they allow themselves to stand authentically in the world, I can only wonder: From whence comes this attachment to suffering? What beliefs hold me back? What patterns drain me? Do I trust the inevitability of success when I say yes to my dharma? Yoga teaches us to ask these questions and to have faith that, if we are on a spiritual path, the time for asking questions will be temporary. The questions will be followed by answers, the answers by action, and the action by growth.

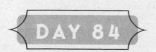

DAY 84

Through spiritual reading, disciples gain communion with the divine power on which their hearts are set.

Yoga Sutras

The fourth *niyama* is *svadhyaya,* which literally means education of the self, or self-study. This observance is most commonly associated with the expectation that the serious yoga student will develop the practice of reading sacred literature. In my own life, this means that I am always reading something by one or another of the writers I consider my spiritual teachers. This is not to say that I don't treat myself to some trashy fiction or a history book—but I stay close to the words of my teachers as well. I read their books over and over again, and as the years go by I find that their lessons are always fresh. This reading practice works both to ground my everyday behavior and to give me insight into new spiritual terrain.

As in every other aspect of the yogic way of life, there is a magic to this process of seeking out and reading those works that speak to our true nature. The words of our teachers slowly work their way into our consciousness. Often we find that statements or concepts that we couldn't understand, or had no use for when we first read them, come alive days or months or even years later, as the circumstances of our lives confirm their messages. There is also magic in the ways in which our teachers eventually speak through us. Our thoughts, words, and deeds are informed by the writings of our teachers. It is a magnificent experience to see the beauty of our teachers' souls become manifest in our own lives, to see the loving hands that have touched us touch others through us. Through spiritual reading we gain communion with the divine power on which our hearts are set.

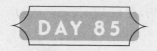

DAY 85

Self-study leads towards the realization of God or communion with one's desired deity.

Yoga Sutras

Despite the fact that our yoga practice has many levels that must be understood before we can grasp its full beauty, the term "self-study" basically says it all. Yoga is the practice of self-awareness. The traditional translations of the sutras describe two aspects of *svadhyaya:* the study of scriptures and the repeating of mantras as a means to commune with, and to draw closer to, your desired deity. B. K. S. Iyengar describes self-study as occurring during asana and *pranayama* practice as well, facilitating the dialogue between the body and the spirit. I would go even further—for earlier in the sutras we are told that everything is a means for self-study, that we are here on earth to learn.

My own practice of self-study is at the core of my spiritual life. I first came to spiritual practice with the sense that I was awakening from a dream. My world had been turned upside down, and spiritual practice was my means for making sense of the strange new land in which I found myself. I had a profound sense of not knowing who I was, what I was, or what I wanted to be. Spiritual practice, for me, has been about answering those questions. I have found that having a job, having roommates, paying taxes, dating, getting married, having in-laws, knowing outlaws, walking the dog, running a yoga studio—in other words, life, all of it—have been the way the universe has chosen to teach me about myself. As far as practice goes, I must be willing to take responsibility for my reactions while I'm on the mat. Why am I annoyed by a particular teacher? Why do I avoid certain postures? What aspect of myself am I not allowing into my consciousness while I hold a posture? What karmic influences are present in my practice? In other words, how am I on autopilot here? How am I turning my practice into just another distraction? To draw nearer to ourselves in this manner is to draw nearer to divinity. There is no separation between us and the rest of the universe. Nor is there an order of importance. There are not big insights and little insights, only insight. To commune with our reality is to commune with the stars, to draw nearer to our desired deity.

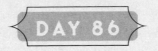

DAY 86

It has been well said that all true art is a contagion of feeling; so that through the true reading of true books we do indeed read ourselves into the spirit of the masters.

Charles Johnston

My life is rich with examples of the power of *svadhyaya* and its myriad effects. Recently I picked up a book by Pema Chodron, who I consider one of my true teachers, in search of material for an upcoming class. As I flipped through the pages, I came upon the suggestion that I should give up hope. According to Chodron, hope is an illusion, a disturbance in our dance with reality. I paused for a second, then moved on, believing that this was not the energy I wanted to bring into my classroom. "Ladies and gentlemen, give up hope!"—no, this was not the direction I wanted to go this morning. But the idea lurked in the corners of my mind.

A few days later it came together for me. For as far back as I could remember, the workweek had been an emotional minefield for me. Mondays were abysmal; Tuesdays were redeemed in the seventies by *Happy Days* but had long since joined Mondays as weekly low points; Wednesdays were neutral at best; Thursdays were bright with promise (we're almost through!); Fridays, a victory walk; Saturdays, confusing; and Sundays were days of mourning as I contemplated beginning the whole cycle all over again. All in all, with this approach, I was able to truly enjoy about two to two and a half days a week. This all changed over the last few years, when I began working seven days a week. These days, I get about two full days off a month. I am in the yoga business, and business is good. I teach a lot of classes, give private instruction, and write about yoga every day. My wife has become a yoga instructor herself so we can spend more time together. Oddly, this relentless schedule has freed me from the lifelong roller-coaster that was the workweek.

When I first began working seven days a week, I went through a period of struggle, grieving for the free time I thought I had lost. But once I got used to my new schedule, it felt remarkably sane. I did not experience any highs and lows during my week. In fact, I lost track of the whole workweek concept. I had given up hope—and this actually felt a lot better than going through the elation and bitterness of my old Monday-through-Friday routine. The truth is, teaching yoga is my dharma. A month straight of doing anything else would send me screaming into unemployment. But I believe I have understood an important teaching and have made it applicable to my life. Giving up hope, I have actually found a new kind of freedom. What's more, I didn't need to understand this immediately; the truth of Pema Chodron's words was slow to dawn. My job is simply to do the work, practice *svadhyaya,* and turn the results of my efforts over to the spirit of the universe.

> The ancient Masters were profound and subtle. Their wisdom was unfathomable. There is no way to describe it; all we can describe is their appearance. They were careful as someone crossing an iced-over stream. Alert as a warrior in enemy territory. Courteous as a guest. Fluid as melting ice. Shapeable as a block of wood. Receptive as a valley. Clear as a glass of water. Do you have the patience to wait till your mud settles and the water is clear? Can you remain unmoving till right action arises by itself? The Master doesn't seek fulfillment. Not seeking, not expecting, she is present and can welcome all things.
>
> Lao-Tzu

Lao-Tzu describes self-study in action. At the core of self-study is nonattachment. If my aim is spiritual health, if I am an artist and my life is my art, then I already have everything I need. Attachment to external circumstances merely holds me back. Nonattachment frees my physical, intellectual, and spiritual powers to such a degree that I can be careful, alert, courteous, fluid, shapable, receptive, and clear. More important, Lao-Tzu is describing the outward appearance of nonattachment. The inward reality of nonattachment is insight. In the clear open space of a nonattached mind, reality can be perceived. The self can be known.

Whenever we find ourselves attached to an idea we have about ourselves or a situation, we are in opposition to self-study. The efforts we make to uphold a certain self-image actually block our insight and thwart our growth. Anxious to uphold our self-image, to acquire an outcome, we cannot wait until our mud settles and the water is clear. Fearful of a negative outcome, we are unable to remain still till right action arises by itself. Self-study represents a profound paradigm shift. It is the moment in our journey when we let go of results and wholeheartedly embrace the process. Once we shift our focus from the results to the process itself, all situations become opportunities. We are present and can welcome all things.

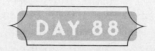

> "Thou knowest I am blind," said the angel, "because mine eyes still retain the light of the Lord's glory, I can perceive nothing else."
>
> Paulo Coelho

Each step forward in our practice is a step inward. To practice yoga is to draw ever closer to the truth. As we learn to relax into our truth moment by moment, breath by breath, posture by posture, the need for pretense starts to fall away. We find that we are shedding the layers of armor we've created to protect the false self we present to the world. But as the armor falls away, we are confronted by the old fears that created the armor in the first place and that have held it in position for so long.

Chances are we will be unaware of the moment when we shed a layer of armor. We may simply wake up one day to find that an old fear has reared its head, or that it seems harder to get to our mat, and harder still to attend to the other aspects of our practice. Suddenly, chocolate chip cookies and Häagen-Dazs are on the menu, gossip fills an hour of the day, an unhealthy relationship appears more attractive. At such times it's important to understand that a resurgence of old behavior often accompanies growth, that such regressions are, in fact, signs that we are drawing nearer to our truth. We see this in the stories of Jesus and the Buddha. Both men were beset by their demons even as they moved unerringly toward their dharma. And both were able to meet their challenges and move on. Their lives are universal examples of the human potential for growth. We all share this potential, and we awaken it each time we practice. Confronting the fears we encounter along the way is an aspect of the practice itself. As the darkness of our fears is dispelled, we become like the angel in Paulo Coelho's tale. Our eyes are filled with the light of love, the love that is ever present beneath all our temporal, earthly loves.

When we do feel lost or uncertain, drifting away from our practice, blocked from our own truth, it helps to remember that darkness and confusion, too, are part of the path. The hero's journey is a journey inward. Yoga is not a workout, it is a work *in*. In the *Tao Te Ching,* we read that the only real movement is return. And this is the point of spiritual practice: to make us teachable, to open our hearts and focus our awareness so that we can know what we already know, and be who we already are.

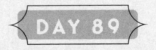

It's hard to read Jung, Eliade, or Cambell, or Huxley without
being permanently affected in our perceptions.

Abraham Maslow

Abraham Maslow brings our attention to a delightful aspect of yoga—the art of staying inspired. Recently I gave a talk to the new teachers at my studio about staying inspired and teaching inspiring classes. The crux of it was that you have to practice every day and you must stay connected to your own sources of inspiration. Whether you are a student or a teacher, expose yourself constantly to those writers, poets, singers, songwriters, movies, actors, yoga teachers, meditation teachers, and anyone else who lights your fire. Just as *tapas* gives us permission to be enthusiastic about our lives, *svadhyaya* gives us permission to stay plugged in. Take yourself out to the workshops, go to the concerts, the museums, the movies. *Svadhyaya* is about connecting to the energy you find healing and inspiring.

At the moment, I happen to be inspired in my teaching and writing by the individuals who created the movie *Gladiator,* so I've watched interviews with the cast, with Hans Zimmer, who wrote the score, and with Ridley Scott, the director. To me, the synergy created by these people is breathtaking; they inspire me with the excellence they were able to achieve. And they remind me of what is possible. Great art and literature, the great texts of all the religions—certainly these have the ability to inspire us; but the person next to you on the bus may motivate you as well. A part of *svadhyaya* is to be open to inspiration where you find it. The carpenter working on the house next door from where I am writing this morning is demonstrating, right in this moment, that our art is possible—and that it is entirely ordinary to allow your art to come to fruition. If your mind is open, it is impossible to be in life without your perceptions being permanently changed.

When the energy simply flows through us, just as it flows
through the grass and the trees and the ravens and the bears
and the moose and the ocean and the rocks, we discover that we
are not solid at all. If we sit still like the mountain Gampo
Lhatse in a hurricane, if we don't protect ourselves from the
trueness and the vividness and the immediacy and the lack of
confirmation of simply being part of life, then we are not this
separate being who has to have things turn out our way.

Pema Chodron

Pema Chodron describes contentment as a means to become whole, a means
for coming into the deep state of connectedness that is yoga. It is a powerful, moving declaration of the truth. And reading these words has changed
my own perceptions. Here is a wonderful example of the need for the practice of *svadhyaya,* or self-study. We simply do not get this sort of information, this kind of deep wisdom, as we move through the day. In fact,
svadhyaya has never been more important than it is now, because a sort of
reverse *svadhyaya* has reached unprecedented power in our time. We spend
our days being bombarded with messages calculated by marketers, politicians, journalists, and the media to create a need for whatever it is they are
selling. This sensory overload is ongoing, and it affects all of us, whether we
watch television or read the newspaper or not. The message we receive
from our culture is: "The world is not safe, you are not safe, you need *X-Y-
or-Z* to be safe. Your life is not enough, you are not enough, you need *X-Y-
or-Z* to be enough."

The opportunity to avail ourselves of better programming could not be
more valuable. As I contend with my own racism and sexism, my own fears,

my own limiting beliefs, I am humbled by the power of the harmful, negative messages that surround me. There are days when I want to check into a spiritual center and never leave. For now, though, I am on a different path. I have chosen to seek my solutions right here, in the midst of daily life. Which is all the more reason to practice *svadhyaya*—to spend time with angels like Pema Chodron.

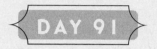

DAY 91

The unconscious wants truth. It ceases to speak to those who want something else more than truth.

Adrienne Rich

Self-study is an aspect of the practice of truthfulness. Any serious attempt at truthfulness requires us to listen deeply to the promptings of our heart. The truth is usually quite simple, but expressing it is another matter. As I bring higher levels of honesty to my everyday interactions, I am struck by the need to sift through layers of illusion, blame, fear, and manipulation to get at what I really need to say in a given situation.

The good news is that truth is music to the soul. There is no end to the soul's ability to bask in the presence of the truth. Millions of people in twelve-step programs sit around in church basements by the hour, listening to one another talk about themselves. It may sound boring, but in fact it is captivating, because the people in those rooms are telling the truth. It is captivating because spending time in the presence of others who are telling the truth inspires us to do the same.

To practice this aspect of self-study, examine the level of truthfulness in your workplace, family, and friendships. How much time do you spend in the presence of people who are telling the truth? How much do you spend with people who are not? What is it like when you hear the truth? What is it like when you do not? What fears keep you from being honest? Is it true that like attracts like? Does honesty beget honesty?

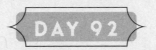

DAY 92

Each body is a universe, as good a universe as you could conceive.

Swami Amar Jyoti

In the West we have cultivated the intelligence of the mind with a passion and a genius that have enabled us to accomplish amazing feats of abstract reasoning. Millions of individuals earn their livings manipulating phenomena that cannot be perceived by the senses. That this is not enough seems unreasonable and suspect. The cultivation of even more wisdom, more intelligence, seems both fantastic and self-indulgent. Nevertheless, millions of us are finding ourselves compelled to explore yet another brave new world, our bodies. The intelligence that is embedded in the cells of a tree and that infuses it with the will to grow tall and strong resides in our cells as well. In yoga we access this intelligence through asana and *pranayama*. The postures and the breath form a bridge between the wisdom of the mind and the wisdom of the body. A divine spark is kindled, and the resulting fire is our spiritual transformation.

An aspect of my practice of *svadhyaya* is humility. In practical terms, that means that I take the time to listen to others who have been where I want to go. I do this through reading, prayer, meditation, attending workshops, and living with my eyes and ears open. Off the mat, I expose myself to wisdom. On the mat, I stand in the presence of the miracle of creation. As I move from downward dog to child pose to tree to fish, I experience first-hand the evolution of consciousness. The wisdom of the tree, the fish, the child, the dog inform my understanding. I can swim like a fish, sleep like a child, abide like a tree, smile with the joy of a dog. An entire universe resonates within me, and the postures and the breath teach me to embrace this universe.

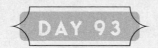

DAY 93

Everything is already OK. The notion strikes us as radical, and it surely is. What it means is that in our essential nature we are already fully awake and enlightened; it means that God is available to us fully in the moment, simply because God is our true nature. We simply have to stop resisting it. There is no distance to travel, nothing special that we have to do to earn God. It's a "done deal."

Stephen Cope

I write in the morning, take a break at midday, and write again in the afternoon. The writing times seem to work for me, but my breaks have been a grab bag. Today, a beautiful July Sunday, my wife and I spent my break in the New England countryside. We had lunch at a restaurant called the Copper Angel, sitting on a deck overlooking a river and a bridge that is famous for being covered in flowers. My wife was charming and the food was fine. Later we found a potter whose work we loved, and I went out to find an ATM so that I could buy my wife a set of matching plates and mugs. As I walked down the sleepy street on the kind of day I dream about, in exactly the place I would want to be on any day, I was uptight and irritable. People and their babies were in my way. The ATM was foolishly located way too far away from the pottery shop. And everything was not already OK.

In a moment of clarity, I asked myself what was causing so much resistance. I couldn't come up with an answer, but I immediately began to relax into my body. Walking in the warmth felt good. My limbs were relaxed and strong. I realized that I did not have to plan the next couple of hours, and as I did, the right plan crystallized in my mind. I began to let go into the afternoon, to just let myself go with the flow. In that moment, the long walk back from the ATM became an opportunity to enjoy the afternoon warmth and the ease of my body. Suddenly I was in heaven and everything was already OK. When we are in hell, we are always that close to heaven, that close to our divinity. We simply have to stop resisting life.

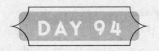

The man who rejects the scriptures, chasing his own desires, cannot attain the goal of true joy or true success.

Bhagavad Gita

In *svadhyaya* the correlation between the study and application of scriptures and spiritual health is spelled out for us. Here, the Bhagavad Gita elaborates: reject the scriptures, chase your own desires, and you will never get where you want to go. OK, so which scriptures? I am Christian, so does that mean I have to read the Bible? What about the Koran? Do I have to believe in one God? The truth is, I don't really know. I can tell you only what has worked for me. In this book I have been at pains to draw quotes from as many different cultures, disciplines, and religions as possible, in order to demonstrate that they are all saying the same thing. The messages are universal.

My own study of "scriptures" has run the entire gamut, from the Bible to Deepak Chopra's *Seven Spiritual Laws of Success*. I am currently reading Stephen King's book on writing, and that falls into my scripture category, too, because I am exposing myself to the truth of someone who has gone deeper in his creative work than I have. Studying scriptures is like poring over maps of territory you are about to explore. It is not a substitute for the exploration itself, but it is still a good idea. Familiarize yourself with the landscape if you want to get to where you're going. The point is, study whatever scriptures help you get where you want to go. If you find something that works, apply yourself to it with *tapas*. Read the same book or passage over and over again, commit it to memory, share it with others, enact it in your life. Travel across time and space, and carry the love embodied in the scriptures in your heart. Share this love with others and you will experience true joy and success.

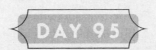

DAY 95

The scriptures dwell in duality. Be beyond all opposites, Arjuna: anchored in the real, and free from all thoughts of wealth and comfort.

Bhagavad Gita

Well, there you go. There really are no magic bullets. We must take the study of scriptures seriously in order to realize the aims of yoga, but we must be beyond them as well, anchored in the real, anchored in our own wisdom. The Buddha said that spiritual practice is like a boat we use to cross the river of suffering. When we get to the other side, we must be willing to get out of the boat. Thus, we must be willing to leave the mat, leave the meditation cushion, and move beyond the scriptures, if that is what is called for by the moment. No aspect of our practice is an end to itself. Practice is merely a means for coming home to our true self.

To place anything above ourselves is to use it as a crutch, a block to real spiritual growth. We all have a tendency to say, "X says that I must do Y, therefore I will do Y." In doing so, though, we absolve ourselves of the responsibility of figuring out for ourselves what is right. And when we don't bother to figure it out, we make a choice not to grow, a choice not to recognize our own innate divinity, our own unique path.

I am pro-choice, but I have witnessed too many women grieving the loss of an aborted child not to have misgivings, not to believe that there has to be a better way. The pain I have witnessed is the real. The political rhetoric on both sides of the issue dwells in duality. To be fully alive, I cannot cling to the comfort provided by the rhetoric on either side. I must be beyond all opposites, anchored in the real, alive to the pain of the pregnant teenager and the pain of the grieving mother. In so doing, I make possible self-study.

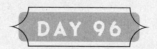

DAY 96

It is called the witness, the consenter, the sustainer, the enjoyer, the great Lord, and also the highest Self, the supreme Person in this body.

Bhagavad Gita

Like the spokes of a wheel leading back to the hub, the practices of yoga bring us back to the self. *Svadhyaya* is self-study, the work we do in an effort to know the divinity that is at our core. But self-study does not take place only behind a desk or in a quiet room; our daily lives are rich with opportunities for practice and discovery. As we move through our days we can either react out of past conditioning or pause and affirm our higher selves. We can allow the power of the universe to flow through us in any given moment on any given day.

For me, the choice is usually to be kind. Most of the time when I find myself blocking that flow, the reason is that I'm withholding myself from a situation. This is one reason teaching yoga is so powerful for me. To teach a yoga class well, the teacher must hold back nothing. The teacher's heart must be entirely open. My greatest challenge is to be open to the ordinary encounter, to not withhold the love in me from the bored or incompetent person behind the counter, the slow driver ahead of me on the country road. Asana are an excellent training ground for this awareness. We can either be in the flow or be in our heads. Moment to moment, our bodies remind us whether we are present or not. In the end it is never about control, it is always about letting go. We are the witness, the consenter, the sustainer, the enjoyer, the great Lord, the light of the world. To access power, we need only surrender to the truth of it. When we are prepared to surrender to our true selves, the need for self-study is at an end.

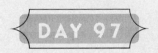

DAY 97

Surrender to God brings perfection in *samadhi*.

Yoga Sutras

The final *niyama* is *isvara-pranidhana,* or surrender to God. When all is said and done, we let go absolutely. I am fascinated by the fact that we have learned how to go about so many things by observing nature. It is said that we learned to hunt by observing packs of wild dogs. What to eat and how to get it, where water is and how to find it, how to fight and how to run—all of these things were taught to us by animal brothers and sisters better equipped than we are. The asana came to us in this manner as well.

My own spiritual journey started long before this notion occurred to me. I came to spirituality by way of human example. Yoga and some reading about Native American culture suggested an alternative, but it was only after my dog came to me as a five-month-old bundle of joy that I really began to get it, to realize that she had much to teach me, if I would only be open to her lessons. I would take her outside and observe her ecstasy. She did not need anything—no sneakers, no scooter, no skis, no SUV; she simply embraced the world and the world embraced her. As this idea moved from my subconscious to my consciousness, I began to consider the spiritual condition of other living beings on the planet. I began to really look at the plants and animals that surround me. What I saw was *samadhi,* complete absorption in the moment, through instinctive, innate faith. In AA they say, "We have resigned from the debating committee." If you want to see what that looks like, gaze out your window. The final *niyama* tells us that we do not have to reinvent the wheel. We simply have to follow suit with every other living being on the planet.

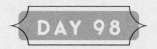

He is love, He is compassion, He is patience, He is tolerance
and peace. . . . He does not try to punish people or send them
to hell. . . . He is clear wisdom who always trusts and believes
that we will return to Him. . . . God always says, "May the
children search for their Father. May they come to Him."
Let us think about this.

His Holiness M. R. Bawa Muhaiyaddeen

My first religion was televised sports. On Saturday afternoons the family would gather round to watch *Wide World of Sports,* which always began with the assurance that we were about to witness "the thrill of victory and the agony of defeat." The "agony of defeat" was dramatically portrayed by a downhill skier hurtling through a violent, heart-wrenching crash. The winners were glorious, and the losers, well, they were losers. Nobody surrendered; you fought to the end. Over and over again, in sport after sport, the fight for survival was ritually depicted. Later, after years of training in the fight for survival, I was playing cards with a group of army officers in an encampment in Germany, temporary quarters where individuals who normally did not cross paths were living on top of one another. A chaplain walked by and my friend said, "Oh, that's Captain White. He believes in God!" We all laughed, as though my friend had said Captain White believed in flying saucers. What could be more ludicrous and irrelevant?

My own fight for survival came to an end when I lost it. Alcohol so debilitated me that even I knew I was through. The resourcefulness and will that had earned me a prep school championship in wrestling and had seen me through army Ranger school was completely outclassed by alcohol. Having nothing else to lose, and a strange sense that there was definitely something to gain, I tried prayer. Prayer worked, immediately and decisively. In the eleven-plus years since I started praying, I have not had a drink, nor have I had a moment's doubt that my prayers have been heard. I have been one of the lucky ones. For most people, faith is a gradual process; for me it happened in the blink of an eye. I was transformed, and all that was needed was the slightest willingness on my part to be transformed. "He is clear wisdom who always trusts and believes that we will return to Him." What was your first religion? What is it now?

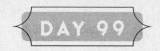

DAY 99

Act as if you trust your God.
Anonymous

A few years back, I met a man whose spirituality has had a lasting impact on me. As a young man he had been a drag queen who favored David Bowie. He was also an alcoholic from an early age and got sober while still quite young. At the time of our meeting, he felt that his sobriety had been split in half by the AIDS epidemic. The first ten years had been a miracle of healing and community; the second ten years had seemed like one long funeral. Sober and monogamous, he had avoided AIDS himself, yet he had experienced its devastation as his entire community was decimated by it. Somehow, the extent of his suffering seemed to bring into sharp relief the depth of his spiritual connection. To be in his presence was to harbor no doubt about the power of a spiritual practice and the sustenance that is to be found in trust and reliance upon God.

For a time we often had coffee together. We both worked second shifts, and our odd schedules were in sync. We were also both in the front lines of the human service industry, after having left more lucrative professions for spiritual reasons. I was having a very hard time in my new field and was spending a good deal of energy feeling sorry for myself. One day, after listening to me rail about the injustices of my employers, he asked if I thought I might someday do a better job. Without hesitation I said, "Yes! I think I will make a great program director someday!"

"Rolf," he said firmly, "go to work today and act in such a way that your coworkers and supervisors would agree with you."

A few days later, when I complained about some other inequity at work, he said, "Rolf, act as if you trust your God." That time, the words stuck. His message to me was always the same: to be spiritual is to act like an adult, to take responsibility for one's actions, to manifest love in one's interactions. I often come to the mat to be comforted. I turn to God as a child to have my pain taken away. There is nothing wrong with this. In fact, seeking comfort is often a necessary first step in summoning the help of a higher power to intervene in a given situation. Comforted, it is then our duty to comfort. Our problem solved, it is up to us to become a part of the solution. There is nothing wrong with coming to our mats to receive. But in order for what we receive there to flourish in our lives, we must take the next step: we must share our gifts with the world.

Try this today in your own practice: As you inhale, draw life energy in. Then, as you exhale, radiate that heart energy out into the world. Both actions must be honored in our spiritual lives. We must ask for help when we need it, and we must give to others as this wise, generous man gave to me. Let us share what we have, be a ray of light in the lives of those around us, and demonstrate that we trust our God.

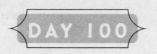

Oh, be swift, my soul, to answer Him! Be jubilant, my feet!

"The Battle Hymn of the Republic"

While vacationing at some hot springs with my wife's family, I received a tip from my father-in-law for withstanding the extremely hot water. As long as I stayed absolutely still, he explained, the water immediately surrounding my body would be cooled, and I would be comfortable. That was all well and good as long as I was still. Every time I moved, though, the heat seemed unbearable again.

Something similar happens as we begin to move in our lives. Practically speaking, the *yamas* and the *niyamas* give us the support we need as we encounter the difficulties of growth. They are actions or choices that accrue us the necessary energy to continue on. You can practice yoga with God or without God. In every translation of the Yoga Sutras we're told that a person can achieve the highest spiritual levels through devotion to God, but it is also acknowledged that this path is not for everyone. We each find spirit in our own way. Devotion itself, however, cannot be sidestepped; it is an essential element of the yogic path.

In class I often suggest that students select something to pay homage to while in *parsvottanasana,* a bowing posture. The energy in the room changes instantly, becoming more deeply focused, as individually and collectively we spend time in the energy of respect. A friend of mine says that he organizes his life around his gratitude to God. Gratitude is the organizing principle, the organizing energy, in his life.

Whether we find profound joy and direction in worshiping God, Allah, the Buddha, nature, human potential, science, or our own higher self makes no difference. What matters is that we embody reverence, that we regularly and consistently bring our attention to the divine.

Martin Luther King Jr.'s life demonstrates the difficulties inherent in making positive change. He could have chosen to stay still, accept the status quo, and be comfortable. Instead, he summoned his faith and moved into hot water, over and over again. Adversity is never comfortable; yet supported by the strength of our principles, we can and do endure it. Borrowing words from a well-known hymn, King's declaration on the statehouse steps in Birmingham defined right attitude: "Be swift, my soul, to answer Him! Be jubilant, my feet!" The power of devotion sustains us as we meet the difficulties inherent in our path. If there is not a dance for joy in your yoga, you can put one there. The final *niyama* is truly a dance for joy. Practice reverence, and experience the joy of devotion.

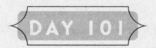

DAY 101

> The real mystic who has spiritual realizations or super conscious experiences becomes extremely interested in his fellow beings as he finds the expression of God in them. A mystic feels the presence of God everywhere and so he takes a loving interest not only in human beings but also in other beings.
>
> Swami Akhilananda

The wise among us do not wait to become real mystics before we begin living this way. A friend of mine has spent the last four or five years addicted to crack cocaine. About nine months ago she went to rehab, and when she got out she joined a church in her neighborhood. The other day she described her practice to me. In the morning, she makes breakfast for her family and prepares her children (who had been cared for during the last few years by her parents) for school. With her husband off to work and the kids out of the house, she spends her days volunteering at the church. Some days she brings food to the elderly, sometimes she assists a mother with her newborn, other times she helps homeless families. She attends regular services at her church and is active in a twelve-step program. She loves her life today, she loves her family and the people in her community, and she loves her God. It really is that simple. Having found the presence of God everywhere, she has also taken a loving interest in all human beings.

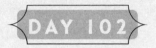

DAY 102

The nature of the universe is such that the ends can never justify the means. On the contrary, the means always determine the end.

Aldous Huxley

Isvara-pranidhana is a statement of the means and the ends. Surrender to God is the means; *samadhi* is the end. In *samadhi* there is no longer a distinction between the person who sees and what is being seen. *Samadhi* is union with the divine, a deep-rooted knowledge that I am that, you are that, all is that, and that is all there is. In *samadhi,* the separation between ourselves and the universe dissolves. This is what it means to surrender to God. Many of my students find this outlandish. They come from this or that religious tradition, this or that experience, and what they have learned makes it impossible for them to believe that the God of their understanding and *samadhi* have anything to do with each other. If you are alienated by the God of your childhood, try coming up with another God.

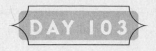

Sell your cleverness and buy bewilderment.

Rumi

My first authentically spiritual practice was saying that I did not know. Long before I was ready to read scriptures or chant mantras, I had to understand that it was OK not to know. I became sober as a military officer, having spent the preceding years pretending to know everything. Despite the fact that I was the only person who believed me, I persisted in my know-it-allness right up until I landed in rehab. Rehab takes the know-it-all right out of you. While I was in rehab, the world changed, and when I got back to my unit there was a war on. I was a military officer in a combat arms unit preparing for war, and I no longer knew everything. In fact, I didn't know anything. I was appalled. Just when my country needed me to have my act together, I was coming to the conclusion that I did not know a thing about life.

What I found was that instead of being a liability, my new awareness was an asset. The truth was, I had never known anything about life in the first place. My newfound cluelessness was actually the beginning of wisdom. Until I was ready to sell my cleverness and buy bewilderment, I could not learn anything. I could not listen to anyone. And I could not be of any real service to anybody. In the frantic weeks while my unit prepared for the Persian Gulf War, I was able to really listen to the men who depended on me. And when I answered their questions, it was with truth. I realized that I had been carrying an immense load on my shoulders, having to know it all, and that without this weight, life was a great deal easier. The enormous amount of energy I had channeled into knowing it all could now be channeled into more productive behavior. I began to form relationships, to learn from others. I began to stand calmly amidst the chaos of life and feel the presence of God. As I emptied my cup, the world flowed in.

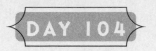

DAY 104

To love another person is to see the face of God.

Victor Hugo

All of our relationships are a reflection of our relationship to God, and our relationship to God is a reflection of all of our relationships. There are times when I see God as I saw my wife the summer we first met, and there are times when I see God as I saw the racist parents throwing stones at children during forced busing in Boston. To understand *isvara-pranidhana,* we must cultivate the same open attention we bring to our asana practice to the forms of love we experience as we move through the day. Just as the many postures are performed by the one body, our many relationships are performed by the one heart.

Bring your attention to the choices you make about love. In infatuation there is abandon. Choice is obscured, and there seems to be only worship. But at some point, does it become real, and do you surrender to love? Consider your long-term relationships, the ones burnished with many warm memories and tarnished by many disappointments. As my life experience deepens, I find over and over again that love is the only answer. Even in my most painful family relationships and friendships—the ones that won't ever go away, whether the person is in my daily life or not—I return again and again to the place of surrender. I do love this person, and I must behave accordingly. It may not be fair, it may not be convenient, but I choose to love anyway. I surrender to my need to love. What is the experience of surrender? Examine this process in your life, and you will see that it extends to your relationship to God. Look deeply into that which you love, and you will see the face of God.

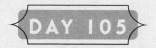

DAY 105

God is love.

I John 4:8

How is love defined in yoga? It is nonharming, honesty, nonstealing, moderation, nonhoarding, purity, contentment, zeal, self-awareness, and surrender. It is being who we were born to be. Love is being who we are. Yoga is a means for eliminating the propensity to be someone else. The aim of yoga is to become still, to learn to reside in our truth. When we are surrendering to God, we are surrendering to the truth in us and the truth in all beings. We are saying yes to love. Begin to notice when you are not saying yes to love. What is your experience of saying no? What is your experience of saying yes? When is it hard to say yes? What would happen if you said yes?

DAY 106

It's so clear that you have to cherish everyone. I think that's what I get from these older black women, that every soul is to be cherished, that every flower is to bloom.

Alice Walker

There is the period during which you undertake the work of *isvara-pranidhana,* the work of devotion to a higher power. It doesn't matter where or how you start; surrendering to God is a process. One day you wake up and you are no longer at the beginning. You've made the change. Your desired deity is at the center of your life. Not only is it at the center of your life, but it is at the center of your friends' lives, and you have supports in place to keep it that way. Now what?

The next step for me has been learning to love the entire universe and everything in it. I had discovered love, but then I had to put love into action. What would that look like? The conclusion I came to was that I had to start treating all God's children the way I would treat the children of an old friend. I have to actively love God's creation, to cherish every soul, every flower. This is why asana comes naturally after *isvara-pranidhana.* In asana practice we learn to cherish each breath, to cherish every cell in our bodies. The time we spend on the mat is love in action.

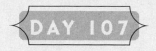

Acting with deep compassion from within my own being,
I dispel all ignorance-born darkness with wisdom's
resplendent light.

Bhagavad Gita

With these words, Krishna describes the internal experience of the work we do with the *yamas* and the *niyamas*. All of this work connects us to the deep compassion that is at our core. We cannot draw nearer to these principles without drawing nearer to our own essence. It is also true that I have not been able to draw nearer to these principles without becoming more aware of all the ways I violate them. My meditation teacher has been at pains to tell me not to make such a big deal of it when I screw up. Picking myself up, dusting myself off, and moving on, I develop the wisdom I need to dispel "ignorance-born darkness."

We have come to the end of the sections on the *yamas* and the *niyamas*. We've covered a lot of ground in a short time, but the work is only beginning. I find that there is so much in these limbs of yoga that when I am working contentment, I tend to forget about nonviolence, and so on. Fortunately, we cannot work on one of the *yamas* or *niyamas* without working on all of them. One way to approach them is to keep one *yama* or *niyama* in mind each day for ten days. At the end, you simply go back to the beginning, *ahimsa,* nonviolence and start over. A simpler way is to choose a *yama* or *niyama* at random and work on it for a while. As you do so, you will see how they all form part of a whole that can be summed by the concept of nonviolence. Embrace the process, let go of the results, and always apply the *yamas* and the *niyamas* on the mat!

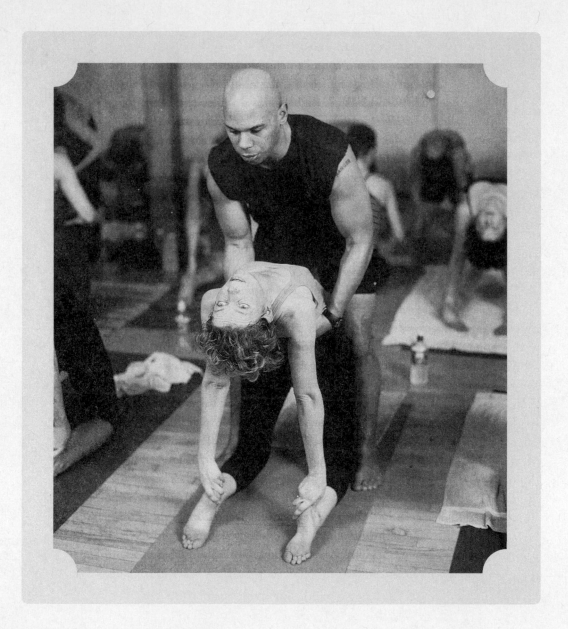

PART THREE

Postures of Yoga,
Postures of Life

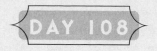

How poor they are that have not patience!
What wound did ever heal but by degrees?

William Shakespeare

The growth we encounter in yoga is dramatic. Physically, mentally, and spiritually we are born anew. I have athletic students for whom the initial effect is mostly spiritual—a whole new world opens before them. For the bad-backers like myself, the initial breakthrough is on the physical plane—one morning we get out of bed without pain. Others find freedom from compulsive worry or obsessive planning to be the first fruits of yoga. But for all of us there is a honeymoon during those first months, as we imagine all our problems evaporating as quickly as the nagging ache in our lower backs. In some ways this honeymoon is very helpful, because it provides much-needed momentum in the difficult process of change.

Inevitably, though, the honeymoon eventually gives way to some issue that simply will not budge. Even in the bloom of our new passion, we realize there are still grave problems at work or at home. Liberated from our obsessive thinking, we discover the depression, grief, or pain that was hidden underneath. As our spines become increasingly flexible, we begin to understand the extent of the physical consequences of decades of compensating for a bad back. Then we embark on a period of reconstruction. And this is where the real work begins.

In *A Course in Miracles,* the adage "Many are called but few are chosen" is used to suggest that although life offers all of us countless opportunities for growth, all too few of us bother to pick up the signals. We don't choose to hear the message. In yoga, the first real setback has the potential to be the last, unless we are willing to persevere with patience.

Preeminent hatha yoga teacher B. K. S. Iyengar calls faith a "yoga vitamin," and patience is truly an unsung aspect of faith. Our practice takes us into the unknown. We deliberately head out into new terrain, off the charts of our familiar world. Such exploration calls for radical faith. But our faith need not be without some underpinning. Shakespeare reminds us that we heal by degrees. We will have bad days and good days, in practice as in life. Sometimes the progress of yesterday seems to have evaporated today. And yet there is always movement. As long as we show up and do the work, healing will happen. This is the message but we must be willing to hear it. We must be prepared to bear witness, patiently, to the degrees by which we move forward. As we learn to celebrate these moments in our practice, we refine our appreciation for subtlety and learn to appreciate growth in those around us as well. And as we practice patience on our mats, our ability to stay with difficult postures—both on and off the mat—grows.

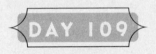

DAY 109

Asana is to be seated in a position which is firm but relaxed.

Yoga Sutras

The earliest visual image we have of asana is an engraving of a person meditating while seated in an advanced posture, the relationship between asana and meditation having been established centuries ago. Some have described the postures, or asana, as preparation for meditation. Others group some asana for meditation and some for physical health. Still others consider the asana to be an end in themselves. I experience them as separate practices, each with its own benefit. I practiced meditation before I practiced asana, but I now see asana as a highly effective way for Americans to prepare themselves for meditation. We are a restless bunch, and a year of steady asana practice lays a solid foundation for the typical American student who wishes to begin meditation. Of course, you should find out what works best for you.

This section deals with the asana, or the work we do on the mat. The emphasis in the above translation of the Yoga Sutras is on the asana being steady and comfortable. The practitioner is to be firm but relaxed. Many new students have trouble with this. They tend to be unstable and panicky. Later on, having bagged a few postures, many students become striving and ambitious. Still later, these same folks become hurt and disillusioned. This is because we tend to approach our postures the way we approach our lives. In our culture, results get all the attention and the process is overlooked. Approach both your life and your postures with an eye to the process, and let go of the results. Stand easy in all the postures of your life, firm but relaxed.

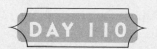

>‹ DAY 110 ›‹

**Like a house protecting one from the heat of the sun,
hatha yoga protects the practitioner.**

Hatha Yoga Pradipika

Having embarked on the magnificent journey called yoga—that is, having embraced the solution—I thought it might be helpful if we established a way to observe the problem at work in our daily lives, so as not to lose sight of our objective. The five afflictions walk with us and talk to us throughout the day, in the voice we have come to call our imagination. What? Our imagination? But that can't be.

Yes, it's true. Having lost our innocence, having found the truth somehow unbearable, we have learned to escape into our imaginations. The fact that we have come by this habit honestly in no way mitigates the fact that it blocks our spiritual growth. Our spirit lives in the moment, and that is where we must be, too, if we are to evolve. For most of us, though, everyday life is a construct of our imaginations.

Caught up in a matrix of resentments and desires, we sleepwalk through our days, imagining positive and negative outcomes for events that will never come to pass. Explore this for yourself. Note the difference in a posture as your mind shifts from the present to your imagination. As you walk through your day, how often do self-doubt, fear, and judgment of others occur in your imagination, and how often do they occur in the present? When you are actually fully present in the moment, feeling your body and hearing the sounds around you, do you experience fear, or peace?

We may live from the inside out in yoga, but we practice from the outside in. We first must break free from the bondage of worldly desires and actions, and then we can begin to connect with the God force within. As lofty as this sounds, it is also quite practical. We cannot connect with anything while caught in the web of imagined realities we call daily life. The first four limbs of yoga systematically deconstruct our tendency to live in our imaginations, protecting us from illusion as a house protects us from the sun.

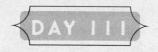

Hatha yoga is a method that will achieve the maximum results
by the minimum expenditure of energy.

Theos Bernard

Everybody seems to feel that yoga is the solution, but what, exactly, is the problem? What is it that makes life so hard? The things over which we feel anguish can actually be summed up pretty quickly. There is the loss of those we love. From the unrequited high school crush to the death of a loved one, loss affects us all. We regret the past and worry about the future. We feel the pain of ill health, betrayal, disappointment. Then there are gross injustices—war, famine, disease, oppression, and death. Most of us don't spend too much time on these big issues, however; it's the day-to-day stuff that brings us down. Why, if I am made in God's image, do I procrastinate, judge others, lose my temper, fail to speak up when I should, speak up when I shouldn't, return the movie late? Why can't I just be perfect? Why can't my partner be perfect? Why are my kids so annoying? What is the deal?

Early in the Yoga Sutras the problem is defined as the five afflictions, or *kleshas:* ignorance, pride, desire, aversion, and fear of death. Under the influence of the five afflictions, we are driven away from our true selves and deeper into disillusion and despair. To put it simply, we seek answers outside ourselves, when in fact the answers lie within. We look out into the material world and identify ourselves with it. Identified with a material world that is completely beyond our control, we are consumed with fear. This fear is at the root of all of our afflictions, our chronic disease, our inability to be happy. The good news is that yoga systematically deconstructs this fear and, with it, the five afflictions. Our true nature is not material but spiritual, and we suffer from mistaken identity. Yoga is a path to our true nature. This

PART THREE

Postures of Yoga

147

truth can be readily tested at the conclusion of any asana practice. The problem is estrangement from self. Check in with yourself at the end of your yoga practice and see if you haven't experienced a miracle of healing. See if you do not feel more at home in your body, more at home in your life, more at home in your spirit. This sense of coming home is real. You have come closer to the truth about yourself, and that is why you feel peace. The rest of this book just brings us that much closer to the truth, that much closer to our home.

Before we go further, though, let's take a look at each of the five afflictions in turn, for only by shining a spotlight on the obstacles in the path can we see the path itself.

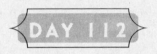

Lack of true knowledge is the source of all pains and sorrows.

Yoga Sutras

The first of the afflictions is *avidya,* or spiritual ignorance, the cause of all the remaining afflictions. The fear that drives us away from ourselves is rooted in our spiritual ignorance—we do not know who we really are. If we did, we would realize that there is nothing to fear. We would know that we are everything we have always hoped we would be but never believed we could be. It is this never believing that is the problem, for with it comes an endless array of compensations. And with each action that stems from this misinformation, we are ensnared more deeply in our illusions.

The good news is that we are who we are. We are an aspect of the divine spirit, and this will always be true. It has always been so and will be so forever more. Our pain is simply feedback from the universe: "No, that's not it; no, that's not it either. Oh yes, you are getting a little warmer, a little warmer. Ooops, you're getting a little colder." Our brothers and sisters who have gone before us have left many road maps to the truth. We sing the truth to one another in pop songs, write it to one another in poems, build statues and cathedrals in honor of it. We scream the truth at one another in heated arguments, whisper it in intimate moments. The truth surrounds us, beguiles us, nourishes and supports us in our darkest hour. The truth lives and is eternal. It is the light, and yoga is about moving toward it.

I believe that those of us who practice yoga have been sent to yoga by our pain. We embarked on this path because we had a hunch that there must be a better way. We have grown tired of our perfectionism, our unhappy relationships with our bodies, our inability to love completely or be loved completely, our endless resentments and sorrows, our sense that we could become greater than we are but that we are somehow blocked. Many of us have had considerable good fortune. We were blessed with the nice smile, the right education, the right opportunities. We may have loving partners, good work, healthy families. Yet we've found that arranging our externals in just the right way doesn't bring us the happiness we hoped it would. The resting place always seems to be just over the next hill. And we have grown tired. We come to yoga in the grip of *avidya*. We come to yoga having forgotten where we come from and who we are. On our mats, we find the truth. We are of God and there are no problems. We are the solution.

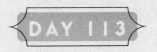

ASANA

> Mistaking the transient for the permanent, the impure for the
> pure, pain for pleasure, and that which is not the self for the
> self: All this is called lack of spiritual knowledge, *avidya*.
>
> Yoga Sutras

According to the Yoga Sutras, *avidya* is the source of all our troubles. Little wonder, then, that Patanjali takes pains to ensure that we are left with no doubt about *avidya's* true nature. My own experience of growing up can be summed up by this sutra. Perhaps yours can be, too. It is as though we grew up in a dark room filled with hot stoves. To make matters worse, there were people in that room trying to get us to touch those hot stoves. Growing up consists of touching one stove after the next as we slowly come to understand the nature of our predicament. At first we simply learn to back off when we start to feel the heat. We also begin to question the voices that are promoting intimacy with hot stoves as the key to right living. Eventually we find that there is someone in that dark room who wants us to turn on the light. Initially we are too busy getting burned to listen, but in some still moment, as we recover from a particularly bad burn, we begin to pay attention to that solitary voice, the voice that is urging us to turn on the light and see for ourselves. Those of us on a spiritual path have entered into a dialogue with that voice. And those who do actually turn on the light can, in turn, become teachers to the rest of us.

The hot stoves are the pain that we mistake for pleasure, the impure that we believe to be pure, the impermanent that we mistake for permanent, the things outside ourselves that we allow to define us. All yoga is saying is what we already know to be true: that materialism is a lie, that we are spiritual beings with spiritual problems, and that we need spiritual solutions. No matter how rich or powerful or impressive we may be, in the end we must all forsake external power and embrace the power within.

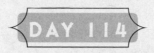

> There's a part of every living thing that wants to become itself. The tadpole into the frog, the chrysalis into the butterfly, a damaged human being into a whole one. That is spirituality.
>
> Ellen Bass

Writer Ellen Bass captures the essence of yoga, the movement of yoga, the inevitability of yoga. Despite the condition of *avidya*, the cloud of unknowing, we are compelled by a sense of a deeper knowing, a higher calling. For many of us, it was early role models—a revered grandmother, a committed high school teacher, a generous mentor—who first embodied our highest aspirations for ourselves. As we grew older, a world of inspiration opened to us. We found direction and beauty at every turn, in the music we listened to, the books we read, the service we performed. But always these sources of inspiration were outside ourselves. We still yearned to become something or someone else.

Yoga encourages us to become ourselves. Charles Johnston, writing about the Yoga Sutras, said, "The steady effort to hold this thought will awaken dormant and unrealized powers." We must cultivate and hold with a steady effort the vision we have for ourselves. And we must start where we are. The path we choose will not necessarily make sense, but we have all experienced the emptiness of "making sense." Now it is time to follow the guidance of our hearts. As Eudora Welty observed, "All serious daring starts from within."

There is a story about Gandhi showing up for a rally where ten thousand people had gathered and, at the last moment, deciding to call it off. His shocked staff insisted that he couldn't call the rally off. What about the ten thousand people? What would they think? What kind of example would he be setting? He replied that he was not there to worry about what ten thousand people thought; he was there to follow the dictates of his conscience. *Avidya* means allowing our choices to be made for us, doubting the truth in our hearts. Grace begins when we dare to allow our prayers to be answered.

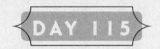

DAY 115

It is better to do your own duty badly, than to perfectly do another's.

Bhagavad Gita

Avidya puts the focus squarely on ourselves. If the root problem is spiritual ignorance, then the solution necessarily entails, as a starting point, getting to know who we are. The genius of yoga is that there are no extenuating circumstances, nothing to wait for, no preconditions to be met. We can begin right now, right where we are. As a friend of mine once said, "The thing about yoga is that you don't have to wait until you've cleaned out the garage to get started."

Yoga provides us with a mirror, so that getting started is not that hard. There are a number of mirrors that you can choose from, but the one most of us use first is the yoga postures themselves, the asana. Breathing in some new rhythm, putting our arms and legs in places they have never been before, sweating in a group of strangers, chafing at the guidance from our teacher, we come to know something of the state we are in. Most of us come to the mat with a mind that is out of control and a poor or nonexistent relationship to our bodies. Nonetheless, we stay with it. We find that amidst the jumble of pride, desire, aversion, and fear, there is a still point, a part of ourselves bearing witness to it all that wants to come back to the next yoga class. Over time, we get to know this witness. It's a bit like being at the bus stop week after week and slowly getting to know the interesting stranger who waits with you at the same stop each day. Amidst the din of our resistance to life, the clamor of our fears, there is a quiet voice whose guidance we learn to listen to and to trust. In the mirror of our yoga postures we begin to see that we are not our pride, our fear, our desire. Over time we find that we are not many other things as well. We make a beginning, we develop a love and respect for the person we meet in the mirror of our yoga practice. We find that we would rather be ourselves, imperfectly, than someone else perfectly.

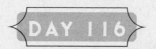

DAY 116

Be still, and know that I am God.

Psalm 46:10

We wake up in yoga as if we were coming out of a dream. We start out befuddled, our identity derived from a lifetime's collection of half-truths and misinformation. "I am thirty-five years old, I come from the Northeast, I am a licensed clinical social worker, and I like to help people." In short, we are defined by externals—by what we do and by all the ways we come up short. Within this worldview, disillusionment and despair are a part of every feeling person's repertoire. Bob Dylan received an Oscar for writing and performing a song with the refrain "I used to care, but times have changed." No doubt about it, *avidya* is a bad place to be, and misery loves company. If we are to derive the truth about ourselves from the media or from the material world, well, perhaps it is best not to care.

The opposite of this unpleasant predicament is *vidya,* or knowledge. In the simplest sense of the word, *vidya* refers to direct knowledge of the soul. In the yogic paradigm, direct knowledge of the soul brings immediate relief from the ceaseless suffering we incur from *avidya.* To better understand this concept, we simply have to reflect on any of a number of moments in our own lives. The moment begins during a fever pitch of obsessive worry, concern, or self-doubt. We are convinced that nothing is more important than the stuck place we find ourselves in. We are defined by our partner, and our partner is leaving. We are defined by our job, and we just lost it. We are defined by the acceptance we receive from a group of friends, and they just blew us off. The slight reed of our self-esteem has collapsed under the strain of our most recent attempt to get something from the outside in order to make us feel OK on the inside. We are betrayed, we are abandoned, our worst fears have been realized, we are unworthy. But—life goes on. We have dinner, talk to a friend, spend some time in our own company. Then there is the moment. For an instant, however brief—on the train to work, on the way to the bathroom in a restaurant, in prayer before bed—we reflect in stillness. We pause and connect to another reality. In this reality there is a sense of timelessness. In this reality, despite our damning circumstances, we suddenly have a feeling that things are going to be all right after all. There is a sense that we are glad to be who we are. The moment passes, but it has left its impression. Life will go on. We will not give up, as we thought we would only minutes or days before. What has happened is that in that brief, still moment, we have had direct knowledge of our soul. We have cut through the mists of our mind and perceived the truth.

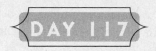

Everything in life is pointing us back to our true nature.

Stephen Cope

A Course in Miracles is a self-study program of spiritual psychotherapy contained in three books. Although the course uses traditional Christian terms, it challenges readers by using them in nontraditional ways, as it seeks to remove "the blocks to the awareness of love's presence which is your natural inheritance." In *A Course in Miracles,* we are reminded that all of humanity's troubles began the moment we perceived ourselves to be separate from God. We all know the story of the fall of Adam and Eve; we left Eden when we lost our sense of oneness with God and each other. But at the very moment the separation occurred, God also created the solution. According to the course, the Holy Ghost came into being to heal the minds of humans who believed that they were separate from God. God gave us free will, so it is possible for us to choose to be misguided. But in God's universe the solution to our suffering became possible the moment we created the cause of our suffering.

In yoga there is a similar relationship between the problem and the solution. The all-pervasive *avidya,* or ignorance, is matched with the eternal *vidya,* or clear seeing. The moment we become willing to believe in a power greater than ourselves, or in a reality more complex than the material world of our own imaginations, we find ourselves to be embraced as intimately by the true as we have embraced the false. The old definitions of time, power, good, and bad are turned inside out and eventually become irrelevant as we realize that our entire belief system has been predicated on false assumptions. Even a hint of the truth has awesome implications.

One of the first ways that I noticed this was in how time was affected in my life. Once I placed my spiritual condition at the top of my list of priorities, I was able to sustain extraordinary spiritual commitments, over long periods of time, with very little effort. In addition, I found that huge shifts and changes could now take place in brief moments of time. Miracles of healing occurred in a matter of months. Financial, professional, and personal circumstances were transformed in the passing of a couple of New England seasons. As we shift our focus from the material to the spiritual, we find that we are truly living on another plane, a plane whose rules can be perceived only by the heart. Once we develop this understanding, the world becomes our classroom. We are always practicing. Some postures we do on the mat, but most we do off the mat. There is really no distinction. Every interaction, each moment, each breath is an opportunity to grow spiritually, to practice yoga. We find that "everything in life is pointing us back to our true nature."

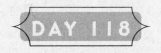

DAY 118

There is the you and the not you. . . .
You are not your thoughts.

The Reverend Jesse Lee Peterson

Until we begin to understand that we are not our thoughts, yoga appears to be advocating a puritanical form of repression. If we are our thoughts, then yoga is simply a perpetual battle between equals. Our thoughts whisper, "Ice cream, ice cream! Oh, wouldn't it be nice to have some ice cream?" And then our thoughts say, "I just ate a good meal, I need time to digest before I go to bed, I will have a better practice in the morning if I do not eat ice cream." Then our thoughts say, "Ice cream, ice cream!" and so on. We have all been there, and this is not a plan for effective living.

The paradigm shift comes on the mat and in meditation, when we discover that there is another player. There is the self who witnesses our thoughts. In Tibetan Buddhism, the analogy is that our mind is the sky and our thoughts are the clouds. The idea is to cultivate the expansive sky and to let go of the limited clouds. As we hold a posture or sit in meditation, we can begin to understand what the Tibetan Buddhists and the Reverend Jesse Peterson are saying. As we hold a posture, an aspect of ourselves is observing and learning, it is growing with our bodies. And yes, there is another aspect of ourselves that is looking at the clock, thinking about all we could do if we left class ten minutes early, adjusting our shorts so we won't look fat, feeling tired or annoyed, exhilarated or unhappy.

Avidya is believing that the endless distracting thoughts are who we are. *Vidya* is the understanding that we are the quiet witness who is present as we hold a posture or sit in meditation. We were never meant to be our thoughts—and that includes those thoughts that are attached to pleasure. To overcome attachment to pleasure, we don't need to repress our reactions to experience; rather, we simply need to systematically develop our relationship with the witness, with the expansive sky. As we hold a posture, it becomes clear that we can cultivate distraction or direction, resistance or peace, a sense of who we are or a sense of who we are not.

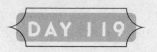

A S A N A

Egoism is the identification of the seer with the instrumental
power of seeing.

Yoga Sutras

Patanjali goes on to point out the second affliction, *asmita*. The definition
of *asmita* is egoism, or sometimes pride. In purely spiritual terms, *asmita* is
the direct result of *avidya*. Having lost track of who we are, we make up a
definition that seems to make sense. *Asmita* is the mistaken belief that our
abilities are who we are, and not a reflection of who we are. It is as though a
lightbulb, having forgotten about electricity, believes that it is light. In a
more worldly sense, *asmita* manifests as the madness of pride, and the despair
that comes from a belief in an isolated self.

Those of us in the United States live upon a segment of the earth whose
resources provide us with enormous material power. The belief that this
power is somehow our fault, rather than a blessing and a responsibility, is
the madness of *asmita*. Conversely, the belief that our material wealth must
be safeguarded from those who share the planet with us arises from the fear
that derives from the isolated self. The isolated self, the rugged individual,
lives in imagined exile from love and safety. *Asmita,* then, is a coin with two
sides. On one side is the sense that we are above everyone; on the other is
the fear that we are beneath everyone. Out of disconnection from self
comes disconnection from others.

As we come to understand *avidya* and *asmita,* we come to understand
how it was that Adam and Eve left the garden of Eden. Falling asleep, we
have a nightmare in which our brothers and sisters are strangers, in which
we are no longer a part of the love that created us. Hungry, tired, and afraid,
we have forgotten who we are, and so we make up a fiction based on our

experience of the dream. This fiction is *asmita*. Convinced that our fiction is truth, we turn away from the garden and from the love we once knew there. And we walk out into the wasteland of our nightmare, a land without safety or love. In conventional time, we have been living this nightmare for many generations. But yoga time is different. In yoga we have never left the garden, we have simply been asleep. Our brothers and sisters have never ceased to be our brothers and sisters, and the love that is our essence is still alive in us. We must simply allow this to be true. As we have believed in the lie of *asmita,* the lie of disconnection, we must now believe in the magnificent reality of spiritual connection.

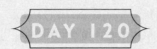

DAY 120

For it is by self-forgetting that one finds.

Prayer of Saint Francis

Over time, the practices of yoga create a state of grace in the practitioner. *Asmita* is the suffering that comes from self-centered fear. As long as we are the unworthy person around whom the world revolves, the pressure is enormous, the fears legion. As yoga refines our natural abilities, releases blocked energy back into our lives, and clears our minds, our hearts become calm and we simply forget our suffering. We go back to our mat day after day, back to the meditation cushion day after day, practice our breathing day after day—and we begin to experience life as an outpouring of grace. My friend Baron Baptiste says that if you practice yoga, your bad habits will drop you. Meditating on the breath, relaxing into a posture, we become open to life, open to our spiritual selves.

Wherever our attention is, that is where we are. As the practices of yoga flourish in our lives, our attention increasingly turns from thoughts that drain our energy to thoughts and situations that uplift us. We find that we have time to appreciate the color of spring flowers, instead of being consumed by nagging doubts or concerns. I recently worked with a woman who mentioned alcohol in every third sentence. Within minutes of meeting her, I realized that she had a drinking problem. In the past, this would have been problematic for me. I would have felt uncomfortable around her, imagining her suffering and feeling repelled by her addiction. On that morning, I felt my reaction come up, and then I watched it dissipate. I didn't have to repress my reaction to this woman; it simply came up and I noted it; this time there was no pull in it. I saw that my typical, conditioned response was a dead end, and that I genuinely preferred to treat her as I would any other person. I no longer had the need or the desire to judge this woman or withhold myself from her in any way. She no longer threatened me. My fear was gone, and what stood before me was a child of God. My yoga practice has reunited me with the aspect of myself that this woman's problem represents. As I have come to accept this part of myself, I am also able to accept this part in other people.

Yoga wears away the self-centered fear that is *asmita*. Each posture, each breath we take, loosens our grip on the life that we have lived and allows for the birth of a new one. Eventually, caught up in the beautiful work of being present for grace, we forget about ourselves, and through self-forgetting we find ourselves.

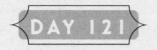

Attachment is that which dwells upon pleasure.

Yoga Sutras

The next two hindrances are *raga* (attachment, desire) and *dvesa* (aversion). Within these are the more specific hindrances of attachment to pleasure, or *sukha,* and aversion to pain, or *duhkha. Sukha* and *duhkha* in themselves are simply natural human reactions. *Sukha* and *duhkha* become *raga* and *dvesa* when attachment is present, for it is in the attachment to pleasure and the aversion to pain that we get into trouble. Attachment to ice cream can lead to obesity, diabetes, heart disease, and death. Aversion to the pain of having a diseased tooth repaired can lead to extreme infection, toxicity, and death. To some degree, attachment to pleasure and aversion to pain can be found at the bottom of most of our difficulties.

The Yoga Sutras address attachment to pleasure first, and certainly this is the more obvious pitfall, the one with which most of us are intimately familiar. As a nation we watched the absurd spectacle of President Clinton sabotaging himself as he was forced to contend with his attachment to Monica Lewinsky. Many of us seem to spend half our lives contending with our attachments to pains that conceal themselves as pleasure.

The five hindrances correspond to the three levels of the brain. *Avidya* and *asmita,* ignorance and pride, come from the cortex, and are experienced as thoughts. *Raga* and *dvesa,* desire and aversion, come from the mammalian brain, and are experienced as emotions. Desire comes from an ancient place in our development. We share this sensation with countless other beings. My dog quivers with desire when she observes a squirrel through the window. A timeless, innate response to experience, desire is a powerful force in our lives. There is nothing to fear in desire; desire is an energy that is an intrinsic, essential aspect of our humanity. The newborn child, Michelangelo's *David,* the thirty thousand people who run the New York marathon each year—all are tributes to the creative power of desire. Yoga is simply asking us to make a friend of this aspect of ourselves and to allow desire to be in our lives as it should be. On the mat we learn to observe our experience, to allow our experience of the moment to arise and to pass away without attachment. *Sukha* and *duhkha,* pleasure and pain, arise and then pass away like drops of rain rolling across the surface of a leaf. We enter a posture we enjoy, experience it fully, then let go and move on to the next one, a posture we like less. We embrace this posture, experience it fully, and then move on. This is yoga.

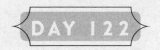

DAY 122

Everything can be "this"; everything can be "that."

Chang Tsu

Desire and aversion arise out of duality. We think, "This is a good outcome, that is a bad outcome," or, "I really want this, I really don't want that." Both in our individual life spans and in our development as a species, we experience the mammalian brain—the black-and-white world of good and bad—before we experience the world of the cortex, the domain beyond duality. As we grow individually and as a species, we come to see the liability in dualistic thinking. Japan and Germany lost World War II. Their industries and much of their infrastructure were destroyed. In the aftermath, the allies helped rebuild these nations with the latest technology. By the end of the twentieth century, both nations had achieved the global prominence they had gone to war to gain. Was losing the war a bad thing, or a good thing? In this circumstance, what is winning and what is losing?

As a younger person, I took refuge in idealism. To the "enemies" of the United States I was counted among the fanatics. I was an Airborne Ranger. I had an office in Germany overlooking an enormous parking lot for U.S. weaponry. For years I looked out my window and watched hundreds of millions of taxpayers' dollars sit in readiness for a war that would never come. The certainties that had once made me feel safe were slowly deconstructed as I reflected on this enormous waste. My life was dedicated to the service of the taxpayers, who, it became clear to me, were being betrayed. And I was a part of the betrayal. Who was right and who was wrong? My life after the army has been spent finding another way of knowing, and learning to trust unknowing.

In order to face *raga,* the attachment to pleasure, in our lives, we must face the certainties in which we have sought refuge. Out of spiritual ignorance is born a compromised sense of self. Out of our compromised sense of self is born attachment to pleasure and aversion to pain. The pleasures we are attached to are merely reflections of our mistaken understanding, our mistaken certainties. Simply imagining direct knowledge of the soul gives us a sense of how absurd most of our fears and desires truly are. Look behind your desire to the reasoning that compels it. Invariably you will find a compromised sense of self. This understanding is yoga. On your mat, watch the shift that takes place as you move toward mastery in a challenging posture. What began as aversion ("I hate that posture") becomes desire ("I am really getting that posture; I hope we go over it in class"). Watch as a posture that was "this" becomes a posture that is "that"—and physically experience the emptiness that resides in the center of duality.

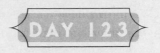

The man whom desires enter as rivers flow into the sea, filled
yet always unmoving—that man finds lasting peace.

Bhagavad Gita

So, the mature yoga student is not at war with desire. She is not vigilantly warding off evil thoughts. Try telling yourself not to think of something for an hour or a day, and you'll see that what we resist persists. Our aim is to be at peace with the world around us. Reactions to experience come up— "Gee, that was nice, wouldn't it be better to have some more?" "I feel flat and empty after that experience; what I need is . . ."—and we let them go as easily as they come. On the mat we often run up against the desire to be doing something else—a different posture, having a cool drink, planning the week. The desire comes up and we let it go.

This becomes life changing when we get to the point where we are unmoved by the fact of the desire as well as the desire itself. Many of us come to a contemplative tradition, like yoga, prepared to let things go. We have already committed to giving up our type-A, work-till-you-drop mentality. The ulcer, the heart attack, the knee surgery, the divorce—something along the way has gotten our attention. And so we attend our first meditation or yoga class and we say, "Right, got it, my thoughts are clouds, I will let them go." And then we go to our mat or our cushion and experience a glimmer of peace—but suddenly, "Damn, I was just thinking about my meeting today, and that's not right. I am supposed to be letting my clouds go. Having clouds is bad. If I were a good yoga student, I wouldn't have clouds." Or worse: "Here I am checking out that guy's butt—and that's not spiritual!" The point is, we are not our thoughts, and so we can let the fact of them go as well. True, you were looking at that guy's butt, but the problem arises when you react to that thought and judge it as a bad one or a good one, rather than as just a meaningless thought. We do want to take our thinking to a higher plane, and that may not include our neighbor's rear end, but we won't ever get there by judging the contents of our random thoughts. Our freedom begins when we accept the fact of our conditioning. We have been conditioned by past actions and experiences to want some things and not want other things. That is simply a fact, just as our thoughts are a fact. We come to the mat thinking we can do certain things and not others. This is past conditioning and it creates desires: "I want to do those postures I know I can do well, or at least not look like a fool trying." Yoga happens when we are unmoved by our conditioning and the desires that come with it.

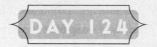

DAY 124

Aversion is that which dwells upon pain.

Yoga Sutras

The next hindrance is *dvesa,* or aversion. Because we have grown up in a predominantly Judeo-Christian culture, the pitfalls of unbridled attachment to pleasure are abundantly clear to most of us long before we hit the yoga mat. The books we read, the movies we watch, the myths that create the fabric of our lives are replete with individuals who get what they deserve in the end, because they coveted or stole, raped or pillaged. The very word "desire" drips with the energy of forbidden fruit. Aversion, on the other hand, is a relatively unknown transgression on the playing fields of Western spirituality. Given that most generations have their defining war, and that we grow up taking stands against a vast array of political ideas and moral wrongdoing, aversion seems quite natural to most of us—certainly not a quality that could get anyone into trouble. After all, fighting Nazis, Communists, cancer, poverty, drugs, high taxes, low tariffs, trusts, and unions—fighting for an idea, a country, or a cause—has always been the American way. How can you have a hero without something or somebody for that hero to fight?

A friend of mine just got back from India. When I ran into her at the store, she was radiant from spending two months at the foot of a mountain in an ashram whose primary teaching was silence. Beaming, she explained that the only thing to do there was to be silent and listen to the wisdom within. In the midst of my hectic day, it sounded like a magnificent idea. In meditation I have found silence to be an indescribably powerful practice. I've also found that I can no more be silent and listen to the wisdom within, while obsessing about one injustice or another, than I can maintain a balancing posture while looking all over the room. There is a truth, we have a soul, we have a spiritual destiny. This destiny is arrived at through stillness. The aim of all of the practices of yoga is to be present in this stillness. Aversion runs counter to stillness. Reacting to experience, whether out of desire or aversion, we are taken out of our center, we lose connection to our intuitive compass.

We all know what this feels like. When I act on my aversion to a situation or person, whether at work or in my family, evolution stops and conflict begins. Evolution takes energy, and aversion is an energy drain. This is nowhere more evident than on the mat. Our resistance to the postures we do not like exhausts us, breaks our concentration, derails our practice. Yoga happens, evolution happens, energy is accrued instead of drained when we are able to see all postures, all situations as the path that leads to our home.

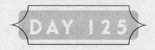

DAY 125

Thinking about sense objects (things we find pleasurable)
will attach you to sense objects; grow attached and you will
become addicted.

Bhagavad Gita

Here we see attachment spelled out for us as a chain of events. Wherever our attention is, that is where we are. Our attention, our awareness, breathes life into that which it rests upon. Place your attention on something, and it grows in your life. Take your attention away from something, and it fades away. Hence the power of asana, the systematic bringing of attention to our bodies, to the state of our minds, to the moment at hand. Alive in the presence of an unwavering attention, our bodies achieve their profound potential. Alive in our unwavering attention, anything can become like the bucket and broom in the tale of the sorcerer's apprentice. Work, money, worry, shopping, exercise, lip balm, Twinkies—the list is endless. None of these items have power in themselves; their power is derived from the power of our attention.

There is a momentum to our habitual thought patterns. Long before we act on an addictive impulse, our attention has given the object of our desire power in our lives. The answer, according to the Yoga Sutras, is to tie your attention to the solution and not the problem. Shift your focus. If you have a bad habit from 6 to 7 P.M., find a good habit with which to replace it. Every day we practice is an opportunity to observe this process. I can view my practice as a tedious obligation and go through my day dreading it. Or I can shift focus and see my time on the mat as an opportunity to experience the power of the universe, to tap into my potential and end the cycle of suffering in my life. The joy of that possibility can imbue my day. In the end, it is all a matter of where I place my attention.

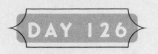

> If one knows what the particular disease is there is the possibil-
> ity of curing it. To know the particular limitation, bondage or
> hindrance of the mind, and to understand it, one must not
> condemn it, one must not say it is right or wrong. One must
> observe it without having an opinion, a prejudice about it—
> which is extraordinarily difficult, because we are brought
> up to condemn.
>
> J. Krishnamurti

Alcoholics Anonymous has arguably one of the most remarkable track records ever compiled in the difficult struggle to alter the course of a human life for the better. By the millions, people have gone to AA, let go of their addictions, found God and meaning in their lives, and moved on. It is an awesome reality. The first step in the process of turning your life around in AA is the admission of powerlessness over your addiction. This admission of powerlessness has been the wellspring from which millions have drawn their strength, and it is also the source of endless controversy. Fortunately, we don't have to debate this issue here. Rather, we can reflect from the side-lines on how AA's first step sheds light on our discussion of a more ancient path. If we were to follow Krishnamurti's advice, and observe without con-demnation, what would that feel like?

By and large, most of us observe our own transgressions—whether they are in the bedroom or in the boardroom—as though we know better, could do better, should do better, will do better next time. As we observe other individuals, companies, political parties, and nations, we tend to bring the same kinds of judgments to bear, expecting different results. In college I wrote a paper about a Central American country in which the north and the south have taken turns oppressing each other for generations. Most of us are all too familiar with such scenarios; it appears to be part of human nature to allow ourselves to stay stuck indefinitely. Caught up in a cycle no less destructive than this small embattled country's, many of us stay stuck by being angry over our anger, sad over our sadness, lying to ourselves about our dishonesty. What would it mean to simply acknowledge our behavior without judgment, without denial, without hedging? Right now, in this moment, can you control your habitual responses to experience? Can any of us not be afraid? Can any of us not know desire? What would be a reasonable first step in forming a healthy relationship to something as fundamentally out of our control as our own deepest desires and aversions? Does an admission of powerlessness appear entirely unwarranted? Could a letting go at that level free us from the fruitless and endless struggle to control the uncontrollable? Could that kind of letting go deliver us to the place where we can begin to work honestly with what is?

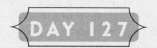

DAY 127

We are tied to what we hate or fear.

Swami Prabhavananda

Our attention can bring alive what we don't want as readily as it can bring alive what we do want. I went to school in Boston during the years of desegregation. Minorities who had previously attended schools in their own neighborhoods were bused to distant schools in an effort to achieve racial parity, and a conflagration ensued. A good portion of white Boston was up in arms, political careers were made by stirring up racial hatred, and hundreds of innocent children suddenly found themselves at the center of an enormous ideological battle. I was twelve and thirteen during the height of the hatred and violence. An implacable bitterness formed in me during those years as I experienced abuse from adults who should have known better. I left Boston as soon as I could and spent ten years traveling and living in different parts of the world. But the bitterness was always with me, and I was convinced it would never change.

Serving in the military in Germany years later, I had a spiritual awakening. One day I lived in a world without God; the next day, God was in the center of my universe. My spiritual growth, and helping others with their spiritual growth, became the priority in my life. Caught up in the wonder of this, I finished my military service, returned to Boston, and moved in with my sister. As it turned out, she was living within a mile of the very school where I had been abused as a child. I found myself walking the same streets, sharing the same bus stop, sitting on the same bus as I had years ago, surrounded once again by the very people who had hated me. The spiritual program I attended had meetings all over the neighborhood. In fact, I became a regular at meetings where twenty to a hundred of my old enemies gathered together to support one another and worship God. It was wonderful. I had shifted focus. Instead of seeing Boston as a place where a deeply troubled people lived restlessly, waiting to inflict some new outrage upon me, I now saw it as just another place where God exists. I found myself falling in love with the city I had fled so bitterly. In the ten years that I've been back in Boston, I have never encountered racism. Instead, I've encountered much love and selflessness. And I've found that the world we live in is a reflection of our hearts.

DAY 128

The desire to cling to life is inherent both in the ignorant and in the learned. This is because the mind retains impressions of the death experience from many previous incarnations.

Yoga Sutras

To the Western reader it appears a little odd that Patanjali felt the need to explain the fear of death. Living in a society in which the preservation of life is a trillion-dollar industry and the worst thing that can happen to anyone is death, it's hard to imagine why anyone would feel the need to tell us why we're afraid to die. Here, more than anywhere else in the Yoga Sutras, we clearly see the cultural difference between East and West. In the Judeo-Christian context, life is a one-shot deal. Within a Hindu context, though, this life is just another episode in a very long series of lives. The extent to which this has been true for the average practitioner of yoga over the ages cannot be overemphasized.

I recently met a retired businessman from India. He was in his late fifties and was traveling from ashram to ashram in the United States. We met at the Kripalu Center in western Massachusetts, where he explained to me that now that he has retired, he is working on his next life. He had devoted the earlier portion of his life to family and business matters; now he intended to spend the last twenty or thirty years of this life securing a good rebirth. The Yoga Sutras were written by a man who inhabited a world that was radically different from ours.

As a Westerner, I have chosen not to spend much time on the metaphysics of the hereafter. At the beginning of my spiritual life, I was surrounded by others who were just starting out, and we all spent a good deal of time debating whether or not there is a God. I decided that I would prefer to live as though there is a God, only to find out that there isn't, rather than to live as though there isn't, only to find out that there is. I take the same stance on the birth/rebirth issue. Who knows? What *is* true is that all the laws of yoga apply in this life. Fearing death hasn't proved helpful to anyone over the entire course of human history. On the other hand, there's a lot to be said in favor of the yogic proposition that we get over our fear of death, our own and others'.

In this life we have been given a series of postures to perform. Death is one of them. Among sober alcoholics there is a beautiful tradition of pointing out, when a fellow traveler passes on, "She died sober." This phrase implies the shift of focus that yoga teaches us. It's not the fact of our death that should concern us. Rather, our focus should be the spiritual condition in which we meet this eventuality.

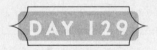

DAY 129

A hundred times a day I remind myself that my life depends on the labors of other men, living and dead, and that I must exert myself in order to give, in measure as I have received, and am still receiving.

Albert Einstein

My first spiritual adviser used the phrase "making your bed" to describe the ongoing work of self-care. The eight limbs are a way to make our bed. They are work orders for living well. Having laid out the means for a good life, Patanjali goes on to define the ends—the *purusartha,* or the four aims of life. Readied for life by our practice, we are able to embrace the *purusartha.*

According to the Yoga Sutras, the four aims of life are *dharma, artha, kama,* and *moksa.* In this instance, *dharma* is the active observance of spiritual discipline. It is the weaving together of the *yamas* and the *niyamas* into a way of life. If *dharma* is the creation of a life in balance on a spiritual plane, then *artha* is the creation of a life in balance on the physical plane. Work, family, money—all are brought into balance and are in keeping with one's spiritual values. *Kama* is enjoyment of the fruits of one's labors. It is not enough just to plant the garden and cultivate it with care; we must set aside time to enjoy it as well. *Moksa* is the final aim of life, liberation. *Dharma, artha,* and *kama* are our actions; in *moksa* we surrender the fruits of our actions to the universe. We let go of everything and hold on to nothing.

We are all performing the *purusartha* in our own ways, just as our parents did and our grandparents before them. We do not need yoga in order to work toward a happy, fulfilled life. Yoga simply gives us an outline. The *purusartha* bring together all the work of this path. They are like the forest, while the individual limbs of yoga are the trees. Use the *purusartha* as a means to keep sight of the forest as you immerse yourself in the trees ahead.

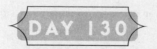

DAY 130

A hundred times a day I remind myself that my life depends on the labors of other men, living and dead, and that I must exert myself in order to give, in measure as I have received, and am still receiving.

Albert Einstein

I think this wisdom from Einstein bears repeating as we discuss *purusartha,* for in this one sentence he manages to address all four aims in life. *Dharma,* the first aim, is the action you take to live your beliefs; it is walking the walk. Einstein says that he has to remind himself a hundred times a day to have the proper perspective. That has been my experience of *dharma*. *Dharma* is not about getting "good," it is about valuing a spiritual choice and doing whatever it takes to bring that choice into your life. Pause for a moment and take an inventory: On what spiritual choices am I acting? On what spiritual choices am I not? In what cases am I willing to do the work, and when am I not? *Dharma* is a reminder that we must be willing to act on our beliefs. It is also the state, the experience, of being in harmony with one's beliefs. Yoga tells us quite plainly that an aim in life is to be one who is doing the work.

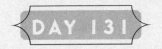

DAY 131

A hundred times a day I remind myself that my life depends on the labors of other men, living and dead, and that I must exert myself in order to give, in measure as I have received, and am still receiving.

Albert Einstein

The second aim in life is *artha,* and Einstein speaks to this as well. *Dharma* is inner harmony, while *artha* is outer harmony. The practice of *artha* is the work we do to remove the blocks to peace in our lives. In my part of the world, I meet many wealthy, successful people who are not happy in their work or in their relationships. This is not *artha*. *Artha* is being in harmony, bringing the *yamas* and *niyamas* into our relationships to work, family, and money in order to create abundance and peace. *Artha* is putting one's spiritual values into practice.

In my own life *artha* has been an opportunity to walk the walk. It has also been a process. For the first few years of my spiritual journey, all I could do was show up for work and try to have a good attitude. Over time, as I have matured, I've slowly created a life that is an expression of my deepest beliefs. I started with just an idea, one priority. For me, that priority was service. I had some ideas about what a life of service would look like, so I worked hard to realize them. Eventually I began to work less, try less, and allow things to happen. I still have my values, my spiritual choice to be of service, but I have let go of the details. Today I simply show up and try to be of service to whoever is put in my path, in whatever capacity the universe chooses.

Examine the fit between your outside and your inside. If there is a gap, make a list of the changes you would like to see happen, create a brief outline of the life you would like to live—and then put it away. Keep the list with you, in your wallet or purse, and update it as necessary, but don't labor over it. Be willing to allow these changes to happen. Don't resist them. Trust that *artha* is a natural by-product of being in the flow of life, giving what you wish to receive.

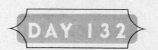

DAY 132

A hundred times a day I remind myself that my life depends on the labors of other men, living and dead, and that I must exert myself in order to give, in measure as I have received, and am still receiving.

Albert Einstein

Read these words, again, and you know that Albert Einstein is grateful. He does not take life for granted. This is *kama*. When we are swept up in the challenges of *dharma* and *artha,* it is easy to become very serious. Wading through our habitual reactions, our fears, our pride, our anger, we can come to see spiritual life as a duty to be endured. *Kama* brings our spiritual work into balance. It is the joy of the journey, the sense of wonder at the symphony that is life.

The foundation of my spiritual life is gratitude. Gratitude is my connection to the real, to the good vibration, to the universe. This is *kama,* and it is my start point. From there, anchored in the real, I can go out into the world mindful of my place in things, aware of my connectedness to all beings, of our interdependence, of our oneness.

Practicing asana, we appreciate the totality of our experience in a posture. Practicing *kama,* we appreciate the totality of our experience.

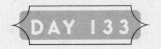

DAY 133

Try to do everything in the world with a mind that lets go. If you let go a little you will have a little peace. If you let go a lot you will have a lot of peace. If you let go completely, you will know complete peace and freedom. Your struggles with the world will have come to an end.

Achaan Chah

Moksa literally means "liberation," to be free. In the flow of our practice, it is the action of letting go. We do our duty, live abundantly, express gratitude, and let go. *Moksa* is the state of nonattachment, the releasing of the fruits of our actions, our efforts, our hopes and dreams. In yogic wisdom, the one thing comes to us as two, and we must learn to accommodate pairs of opposites: desire and aversion, love and hate, man and woman, simplicity and paradox. In the *purusartha,* we are presented with two things—committed action and nonattachment—that we enact as one. All of the passion we bring to the work we do in *dharma* and *artha* is for naught without the dispassion of *moksa.* Conversely, the open space of *moksa* has no meaning without the focus and drive of *dharma* and *artha.*

At the end of each of my classes, I say, "We show up, burn brightly, live passionately, hold nothing back, and when the moment is over, when our work is done, we step back and let go." Carry the two things in your heart, practice them as one, and your struggles with the world will come to an end.

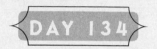

The word yoga signifies the means to realization of one's
true nature.

Sri K. Pattabhi Jois

The Yoga Sutras are a road map to the self. Within the Yoga Sutras we discover both the problem and the solution. The four aims of life are the arenas in which we enact our return to the self. The eight limbs of yoga are the day-to-day choices and actions that we can take, within those arenas, to connect to the self. See and understand the *purusartha* and the eight limbs as two, but practice them as one. Carry a sense of the big picture into your day-to-day actions, and maintain a sense of the particulars in your vision of the whole.

For example, nonviolence is an aspect of the eight limbs; it is a particular. Where do we practice nonviolence? We enact it in our *dharma,* our relationship to ourselves; we enact it in our *artha,* our relationships with others; we enact it in our *kama,* our attitude; and we enact it in our *moksa,* our relationship to the universe. How do we practice *artha,* the practice of abundant living? We apply the eight limbs of yoga to our daily affairs. Every moment becomes yoga, every moment becomes a step on the path back to our true nature.

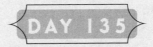

DAY 135

Out beyond ideas of wrongdoing and rightdoing, there is a field. Meet me there.

Rumi

Over the millennia, yoga has traveled between two opposing views of spiritual practice. In one view, the world is flawed, and the individual, an aspect of a flawed world, is flawed—and yoga practice is meant to transcend our flawed nature. In the other, everything is already OK—and our practice is meant to remove our blocks to seeing this truth. Now, this may seem like semantics, but in fact nothing could be more important to sort out before beginning serious spiritual practice.

Patanjali's Yoga Sutras come from a time when yoga was practiced to transcend humanity's debased condition. Note the wording of the following sutra: "Pleasure leads to desire and emotional attachment." Bad pleasure. The world is split into good and bad. The sutras have remained relevant because they speak the truth. What is in question is how one chooses to use the truth. Are the sutras a means of escaping a debased world, or are they a set of instructions for becoming fully alive in *this* lifetime?

I am of the mind that everything is already OK. For me, the sutras are an arrow pointing to the divinity within all of us. It is a given that in asana practice we do not disavow any aspect of our experience or our physicality.

Rather, we progressively embrace what is real for us, so that we may find health and harmony. Why would this not also be true concerning every other aspect of ourselves? As you go deeper into the sutras, spending time with superlatives and ideals, remember that you are doing this study in order to remember yourself, to come home to all of *you*. Only after we get beyond ideas of right and wrong can we truly begin the practice of yoga.

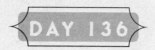

DAY 136

You must learn to be still in the midst of activity and to be
vibrantly alive in repose.

Indira Gandhi

For most of us, the asana are a long walk back. I spent years on the mat thinking this was not so for me, because as an athlete I had had a very physical past. As my practice has deepened, though, I've become aware that I have had to start where everyone starts, with my relationship to God, my body, and to everything else. The fear that separates me from myself, from God, and from others had separated me from my body as well.

I realized the truth of this when I finally got to the point where my practice was no longer about results. As long as I was practicing to get somewhere, I was not able to understand where I was. For me, the breakthrough came while I was teaching, and watching my students struggle with this on their mats. As I taught others to become still, my teachings began to seep into my own awareness. I began to see that my practice was just another goal-driven exercise, and not what it was meant to be—the exploration of stillness in action.

The long walk back has been about experiencing where I am. It's about remembering my feet in a posture where my focus is elsewhere, learning to delight in the how and when as opposed to the why. The asana are a road map to our true natures. In T. E. White's children's classic *The Once and Future King,* Merlin educates the young Arthur by turning him into one creature after another, so that he may better understand the various aspects of his own nature. This is the journey of the asana. We learn to be calm and still in action, vibrantly alive in stillness.

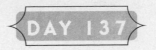

DAY 137

Hell is the place where nothing connects.

T. S. Eliot

Yoga practice gives us a daily experience of the power of connection. We come to the mat fresh from a culture that teaches us that safety is found in separation and disconnection. If we believe that what happens in one school system doesn't affect another school system; if we believe that what happens to one gender doesn't affect the other; if we believe that what happens in one part of the world doesn't affect the rest of the world, then we can convince ourselves that we are safe. But to rely on disconnection for protection is to rely on falsehood. As Martin Luther King Jr. said, "Truth pressed to the earth will rise again."

Deep within ourselves, we know the truth. We know that we are all connected, that we are part of something larger than ourselves. But our unwillingness to honor that connection creates intolerable tension. We all carry this tension within us to some degree. When we step onto our mats, that tension is manifest in our relationships with our bodies. The body at the beginning of practice is a catalogue of inadequacies: "My shoulder is hurting today." "I haven't been getting enough sleep." "My legs are really tight." "I haven't been here for two weeks and I am really out of shape." We arrive on our mats with devalued bodies.

A half hour into class, I pause and invite my students to take a moment to connect to the improved state of their bodies. Miraculously, the sack of potatoes they dragged into the studio has been transformed into an alive, responsive, sensuous being. Their bodies have not changed; it is their experience of their bodies that has changed. Their practice has broken through the layers of falsehood, the sense of disconnection that formed in between classes.

As we practice yoga, the intelligence of our minds enters into an ancient dance with the intelligence of our bodies. We become integrated once again. We experience the power of connection.

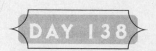

DAY 138

Asana is perfect firmness of body, steadiness of intelligence, and benevolence of spirit.

Yoga Sutras

I have chosen to use a couple of different translations of the two sutras devoted to asana in order to better capture the essence of the sutras' wisdom concerning yoga postures. In this translation we get a better sense of the aims of asana as a practice. Asana are described as improving the body, mind, and spirit. This is news to no one who has had the fortitude to read this far, but it is nice to see that things haven't changed all that much in the last twenty-five hundred years.

Perfect firmness of body, steadiness of intelligence, and benevolence of spirit—that sounds great, but how do I get it? Stephen King says, "Writing equals ass in chair." I would go on to say that asana equals feet on mat.

We encounter our first obstacle to asana practice off the mat—in the form of our endless array of reasons for not practicing today. I generally practice first thing in the morning for just that reason. As the day goes on, I am at increased risk of talking myself out of it. I know all the excuses and then some. And so I tell my students: Plan your week around your practice sessions; develop yoga buddies and make yoga dates; do a little yoga a lot, instead of doing a lot a little. Apply the *yamas* and the *niyamas* on the mat. Buy some cool yoga clothes, get the props you need, buy a good mat, make it fun. Go to weekend workshops if you can, take a yoga vacation. You don't need to make yoga practice your life, but do make it a part of your life. Give the opportunity you have been given the respect that it is due.

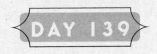

DAY 139

For those who have come to grow, the whole world is a garden.
For those who have come to learn, the whole world is a
university. For those who have come to know God,
the whole world is a prayer mat.

M. R. Bawa Muhaiyaddeen

Relax, and take this in before you practice today. Breathe into these words, this idea. Feel the difference. Most of the time, when I come to the mat, the whole world is a place to confirm my low self-esteem. I come to the mat to strive, to control, to win. Coming to the mat to win, I lose. What if I came to the mat to grow, to learn, and to know God?

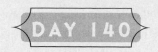

The ego asks a thousand questions for which there are no answers.

A Course in Miracles

We fear everything: success, failure, love, loss, child rearing, childlessness, money, poverty . . . The list is endless. And we bring our most cherished fears with us when we first step onto a yoga mat. We may be worried about failure or disappointment; we may fear the spiritual trappings of yoga, the weirdness of it all; we may be wary of the stranger breathing deeply on her mat to the left, or of the hairy guy standing on his head to the right. Some fears are more personal: fear of reinjuring a vulnerable muscle ("Ah, I thought you should know I had this shoulder operated on fifteen years ago; is that OK?"), fear of commitment ("I have an appointment next week; will that be all right?"), fear of the unknown. Some students fear taking off their socks.

In *A Course in Miracles* we are told, "The ego asks a thousand questions for which there are no answers." In other words, either we can allow ourselves to be continually drained and distracted by a plague of doubts and questions or we can simply choose to apply ourselves to the task at hand. The work I do on my yoga mat requires all of me. If my mind is consumed with doubt, judgment, and self-criticism, then I am not doing yoga; it's that simple.

A friend of mine was deep in a funk, feeling overwhelmed by life, when he ran into his yoga teacher. My friend ran his list of woes past his teacher, who replied mildly, "Whenever I find my plate that full, I just believe that everything is going to work out." So can you. Faith is a choice that is available to us all, at any moment, and it supports us under pressure far more effectively than our own inner debating committee. Today, see what happens when you keep it simple: let go of the questions, set aside the fears, and remember that things will work out. Now breathe, smile, and put one foot in front of the other.

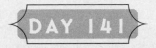

Eighty percent of success is showing up.

Woody Allen

I begin private teaching sessions with a breakdown of what I am trying to accomplish in class at a physical level: strength, cardiovascular health, flexibility, balance, and coordination. As soon as I say the word "coordination," many students wince. Then I tell the story of my wife, whose background has much in common with that of many yoga students I know.

Born into a family of writers and intellectuals whose athletic pursuits were limited to watching basketball on TV and dodging cabs during trips to Manhattan, my wife grew up assured of her identity: klutz. In high school, responding more to her amorous longings than to a desire for physical activity, she roused herself from her books and managed the boys' volleyball team. This brush with athleticism constituted her entire experience with organized sports before yoga.

As a young adult, her experiences confirmed what she had known all her life—she couldn't count on her body to see her through in any situation. On an Outward Bound trip, after days of training in the use of an ice pick to arrest a fall, she slipped and began a precipitous slide down the side of a mountain. Reacting quickly, she hurled her ice pick into the void and would have fallen, had not another climber caught her as she slid by. On a bike trip through Vermont she accidentally knocked two expensive road bikes over the edge of a second-story landing. When friends climbed over a fence on a hike, she stalked off to find some way around the barrier, offended by her companions' insensitivity—they *knew* she could not be expected to climb fences!

Nevertheless, she began to take yoga classes. Soon she was going to class regularly, and to her surprise, she discovered that she liked it. Yoga felt safe and unthreatening; there was no team to let down, no gear to master. What's more, yoga made her feel somehow lighter, less anxious. And as the months passed, she noticed something else, too. When keys were thrown to her, she began to catch them. Once, when she became trapped in the alley behind her apartment building, she climbed a fence, a tree, and a shed in order to make her escape. Today, people often approach her after class to compliment her on her exceptional grace, and she is now an accomplished yoga teacher herself. This ugly duckling has become a swan.

Many people come to yoga having never received a bit of validation for their physical abilities. While those around them are called athletes, they are called other things. The labels become internalized, and eventually a sad thing happens. The "klutz" simply gives up on her or his body, and the negative belief becomes the reality.

I share this story as a reminder that once we commit ourselves to any sort of physical discipline, change is not only possible, it is inevitable. Life is not static. We do not have to accept the pronouncements made upon us twenty, thirty, forty years ago. Coordination, like any other skill, must be learned, refined, honed, and practiced, and that is just what we are doing on the yoga mat. Woody Allen says that most of success is really about showing up. Certainly this is true of coordination as well. So come into the moment, let go of the past, free your body, free your mind, free your heart—and allow grace to happen.

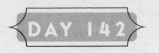

The first problem for all of us, men and women, is not to learn,
but to unlearn.

Gloria Steinem

Every time I encounter a new posture, these words come to mind. Shaking and frustrated as I attempt what those around me can already do (with what often appears to be an excess of perkiness), I am confronted with yet another omission in my planning. Somewhere along the line, I must have said, "Nope, I'll not be needing strength in that area, I'll just bypass it," or, "Gee, I want to run a marathon, but let's not ask my lower back how it feels about it." At some point I apparently told myself, "Men walk like this, sit like this, etc., etc." At a certain time in my life I even convinced myself, "Sports injuries are cool. They are proof of valor." And it all comes back to me in asana practice. Karma is nowhere more clearly demonstrated than on our mats.

The trick is to see the opportunity in our discomfort. We can simply nurse our hurt pride and vow that the South will rise again, or we can see the situation as a good time to get rid of some excess baggage. So do we bring the *yamas* and *niyamas* onto our mats, with nonviolence and surrender guiding us into the posture, and moderation guiding us out. *Tapas* in the middle of practice, contentment at the end. Nonhoarding teaching us to let go of stuff we no longer need. The *yamas* and the *niyamas* stripping away what has to be unlearned, emptying our cup of the past, so that we can fill it in the present.

DAY 143

Society does not want individuals who are alert, keen, revolutionary, because such individuals will not fit into the established social pattern and they may break it up. That is why society seeks to hold your mind in its pattern, and why your so-called education encourages you to imitate, to follow, to conform.

J. Krishnamurti

I am not in a position to comment on your education. Mine was a mixed bag. On the whole it was helpful. Math in particular, though I found it loathsome at the time, sharpened my wits. History taught me to love and respect the beauty of our collective experience. My graduate program in social work helped me see the extent to which I turned a blind eye to the suffering around me. None of it, however, taught me that the love I seek is my own. I did not learn in school that the deep longing I have for this or that outcome is actually the longing I have to be at peace with myself. This information was not in any classroom I ever entered; rather, it was passed on to me by the sages I encountered later, and by every person who has spoken to me honestly. This wisdom is in the smile in my dog's eye, it is the very music of the earth, the resounding truth of the ages—and it can only be heard when we are still. I share Krishnamurti's words with you not to cast aspersions on your education, but to remind you that there is another education waiting for you, and that the teacher will be your heart.

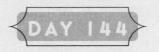

The master gives himself up to whatever the moment brings.

Lao-Tzu

The fall of 1990 was an extraordinary time to be a young person in Germany. The weather was magnificent; the Berlin Wall had come down the year before; the Cold War was a thing of the past. Germany had won the World Cup soccer tournament that spring and I had been in the country just long enough to share the pride, elation, and astonishment of the German people at this miraculous event. Now my time as a U.S. serviceman in Germany was coming to a close and I was savoring my last months in Europe.

Early on a beautiful September morning I went for a run through the pastures and farmlands that surrounded my base. Afterward, I showered and went next door, into my boss's office, to lace up my boots and hear the plans for the day. Major Sitnick was the kind of person I felt most privileged to meet in the army—exceedingly tough, and kindhearted at the same time. To be in his company at the beginning of a day was a particular treat. As it turned out, he had spent the previous evening with his brother, who was staying at a nearby air force base on his way to Saudi Arabia. His brother had informed him that our unit was definitely going to Saudi as well, and that this meant we were preparing for a ground war.

I sat in his office on that beautiful autumn morning and learned that my life and the lives of everybody I worked with were in harm's way. Suddenly my entire world shifted in the space of a second. Major Sitnick read the dismay in my face. "Rolf," he said, looking straight into my eyes, "you have to take the good with the bad."

I knew he was not being glib or cavalier; he had been in combat already and harbored no illusions. He was a kind man and he was helping me to understand the nature of adult life. We set upon a course, and then we must be prepared to take the good with the bad. It is through the acceptance of difficulty that we gain mastery. This worldly older man had learned to embrace good fortune and bad as the same, and so was able to be true both to his vocation and to the people in his life. His example remains with me to this day, as fresh and clear as that crystalline morning.

As I take on the challenges of my yoga practice I am supported by his example. There have been good days and bad days, but I do not expect my practice to be other than life itself. With this attitude I endure and continue to realize my goals. And as a teacher I am able to be of service to others. Van Morrison wrote, "Let me hold to the truth in the darkest hour, let me sing in the glory of the Lord." We can do both, as we practice yoga and as we practice life, learning to give ourselves up to whatever the moment brings.

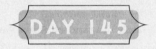

DAY 145

Perfection in an *asana* is achieved when the effort to perform it becomes effortless and the infinite being within is reached.

Yoga Sutras

Although Patanjali wrote 196 sutras concerning yoga, only three of them pertain exclusively to the asana. The first concerns the means—firm, relaxed postures; the second concerns the end—effortless oneness with what is. The sutra above speaks to the first stumbling block most of us encounter in our practice: we try too hard. Despite the fact that all of us have achieved effortless mastery in many areas of our lives, we come to yoga with cultural baggage that says that we are not enough and never will be. We must improve, we must pull ourselves up by our bootstraps, we must try harder and make some progress. With more effort, we think, and a little more strain, we will get more out of the posture. The mistake is believing that we can get where we are going through effort.

Patanjali defines success as effortlessness. Floating in the center of our postures, the center of our experience, we succeed by moving into harmony with the moment, our limbs, our breath, our awareness. Note your tendency to try too hard. Note your impulse to push past the point in which harmony is possible. Note what is keeping you from backing off and simply holding the posture at a point in which integrated experience is possible. Make effortlessness your aim.

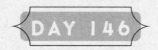

DAY 146

> While performing *asana*, the student's body assumes numerous forms of life found in creation, and he learns that in all these there breathes the same universal spirit—the spirit of God.
>
> B. K. S. Iyengar

As a graduate student I spent a fair amount of time discussing the subconscious. As far as I can tell, though, no one has actually found one. There are none in captivity, and no plans that I know of to catch one. My own understanding of it is incomplete. I say this because whether we understand the concept of the subconscious or not, anyone who has practiced yoga will agree that as the mind quiets, insight develops. The quieting of the mind gains us access to a parallel intelligence. And for want of a better term, we call this intelligence the subconscious. To gain access to this parallel intelligence, we need only apply ourselves to our practice. Control of the breath and the limbs will eventually quiet the mind. In the absence of distraction, we connect to ourselves as an integrated whole.

One aspect of that whole is the infinite creativity of the subconscious. There is a parallel creative process at work in the body. As Mr. Iyengar so eloquently puts it, our bodies contain within them the entire experience of evolution. Our DNA attests to this fact. The mind must become still for the subconscious to come to the fore. The body, however, must simply become at peace to access the wisdom of its cells. The body can be at peace in movement or stillness. If we are practicing with a mind that has let go and a heart that is open, efficiency, and then grace, overtakes our movements. When we are no longer attached to the outcome of our efforts, the intelligence of the mind no longer overrules the wisdom of the body. Then, whether we are moving or still, we have accessed the power of creation. In some moments our bodies spiral into postures like a vine twisting up a trellis. In others, our bodies undulate through movements like a fish swimming through the ocean.

To clear space for such creative expression to occur, however, we must approach our mats with the same intentionality that we would bring to a meditation cushion. We must see that our movements, like the quieting of the mind, have the potential to access an intelligence that has not been available to us. Connection to this intelligence, the wisdom of evolution, will gradually deepen as we cultivate it day after day in our practice. How we move, how we eat, sleep, make love, live, and die will become consciously informed by the divinity of the innumerable beings who have gone before us.

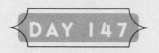

DAY 147

Becoming human means discovering our fullness
and learning to live from it.

John Welwood

Bring your all to your practice. Do not use it as a means to control your weight, or your appearance, or the effects of aging, or anything else. Let your practice be a means to discover your fullness. Be vulnerable, be sad, be happy, be mad, but be there. Just let it happen. Life is about giving, and through giving we receive everything that we need. Let your practice be about giving—give of your heart, give of your spirit, give of your virtue. As Gandhi said, "Be the change you want to see in the world."

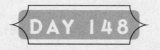

DAY 148

Stay in the center of the circle
and let all things take their course.

Lao-Tzu

It is early October, and the leaves are ablaze with color. After a week of work in the city, my wife and I feel liberated—we are walking in the woods, hearts open to this glorious day, savoring the fleeting grandeur of fall in New England. Even our dog, who has just finished a six-week convalescence from a serious injury, seems to sense her good fortune as she bounds ahead through the leaves, happy to be alive on this day.

Strolling along through the dappled sunlight under a canopy of trees, I am struck by the way the forest reminds us that the seasons are both temporary and eternal. A prematurely bare tree alongside the path reminds me that, although winter will soon come, the trees in these woods will have leaves again. A deserted dock on a deep-woods pond beckons with memories of the hot summer days just past. It is easy to be fully present on this still, clear day—even the waning sunshine suggests the transitory nature of our own existence. We must live it, bask in it, while we may, here on earth for our own brief seasons, and then let go, making room for new lives to be born. There is some sadness in these reflections, yet they bring their own measure of serenity as well. This is how life is, how it has always been. There is a paradox in the wisdom of the forest. This cycle of life, death, and rebirth has been going on since the beginning of time. The timelessness of it fills me with awe.

In the midst of an urban winter, though, I have no such perspective. Emerging from my ever-shrinking apartment into a frozen landscape, I am certain that winter will never end. Spring will not come this year, and I might as well get used to it. Disconnected from nature, caught up in the world of work and the vagaries of daily life, I miss nature's subtle messages, the daily variations in earth and sky that signal the slow turning of the seasons. In the city I live in my head, noticing little; I forget that I ever knew anything else.

There is intelligence in nature that brings balance and harmony to the mind, heart, and soul. When we are disconnected from this intelligence we slowly drift out of balance. This is also true of our yoga practice. Yoga brings us from disconnection and fear to connection and love. Through our practice the intelligence of our minds connects with, is infused with, and joins the wisdom of our bodies. Our bodies contain the wisdom of the forest, the beauty of a sunrise, the peace of a summer evening. It is this force, this power, this energy that we find on our mats. In the presence of the millions of miracles contained in our bodies, we are grounded in the truth. And, like the city dweller rushing through crowded streets, who forgets he ever knew the wisdom of the forest, we can forget we ever knew the wisdom of our yoga. It is essential to make our practice a priority. Accord your practice the importance it is due. Lao-Tzu wrote, "Stay in the center of the circle and let all things take their course." Our practice is the way into the center of the circle.

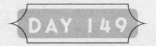

DAY 149

Posture becomes firm and relaxed through control of the natural tendencies of the body, and through meditation on the infinite.

Yoga Sutras

Here is another translation of the second sutra on asana. We are told to control our natural tendencies and to meditate on the infinite. Well and good. But how does that help us during a sleepy Monday morning at the old yoga studio? In my own practice, I've taken this sutra as encouragement to develop new habits and to keep my eyes on the prize.

I recently attended a workshop given by senior Kripalu yoga teacher Stephen Cope, in which he advised us to "make a friend of boredom." For me, this falls into the category of developing new habits. On that sleepy Monday morning at the studio, one of the obstacles to practice is boredom. In general, boredom is a crushing foe to my enjoyment of practice. I can trudge through my postures in spite of boredom, but my boredom remains an affliction. Stephen suggests that we develop a new habit around boredom. Instead of reacting to it or supressing it, we can simply include it in our process. In so doing, I am taking a step back. I am shifting my focus from the problem to the solution. I am meditating on the infinite. Each obstacle we encounter to practice contains within it a similar opportunity to see the world with fresh eyes.

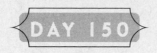

Let the beauty that you love be what you do.

Rumi

In class I often repeat this quote after talking about the concept of *dharma*. In Buddhist philosophy, *dharma* refers to the ultimate law in all things. But it also concerns an individual's right conduct in conformity with this law. On the practical level, *dharma* is the recognition that each of us is born with unique gifts, and that it is our path to discover these gifts and share them with others. In sharing our gifts we live most fully, perform maximal service to those around us, and empower them to live out their *dharma*. It is a beautiful notion, and quite provocative to consider in the context of a yoga class, but invariably someone comes up to me after class and asks, "What if you have no idea what you want to do?"

More often than not, this question is asked with real pain. Most of us live in dread of missing our own lives. My answer is twofold. First I ask, "What would you do if you had all the time and all the money in the world?" This is a very clarifying question, and I often ask it of myself as well, just to be sure I am on the right track in my own life. But if this question doesn't feel helpful, I ask, "What do you do in your free time, when no one is watching?"

Chances are we already know what makes our hearts sing, we already know the beauty that we love. The problem is that we have been trained to believe that the power to fuel our dreams lies outside ourselves, that our unique gifts must be described in a preexisting job description for them to be legitimate. It was a real breakthrough for me when I stood in my bedroom one day, smiled to myself, and said, "I guess my *dharma* won't be spelled out for me in a want ad section or a grad school catalogue."

Dharma is a gift from God inscribed upon the heart. Once we begin to recognize it, we realize that it has been with us all our lives. *Dharma* is what makes you *you*. I see my *dharma* in my yearning for expression, my love for interaction, my passion for details. What is yours?

I read once that if we look closely at a stone we can see traces of the fires that created it, and if we look into a person's eyes we can see reflections of all of the eyes they have looked into with love. So it is with our *dharma*. As we reflect on the millions of smiles of our lifetimes, we see our *dharma* looking back at us with love.

Our practice readies our bodies, our hearts, and our minds for the deep work of living our dreams. As we inhale, we prepare; as we exhale, we deepen the posture. Coming to the mat, we prepare; going forth into our lives, we shine. Our practice is an inhalation, our *dharma* is an exhalation.

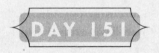

DAY 151

I thank God for my handicaps, for through them
I have found myself, my work, and my God.

Helen Keller

A couple of thousand people come to my studio every week, and each and every one of them is moving slowly toward this understanding of the difficulties in their lives. It is a magnificent thing to watch. This person is going through a divorce, that one has a chronic illness, this one an addiction. My students come to me and tell me what is wrong, and what they are doing about it. Over time, I get to watch what happens. What happens is that they mature.

I am coming to believe that the aim of spiritual practice in our time is maturity. All of the workshops, all of the hours on the mat or the cushion, all of the study and reflection and effort appear to be devoted to growing up, in the true sense of the word. We want to be dependable and wise, loving and brave. We want to abide calmly, see clearly, and be of service. It is as though we are all working really hard to become good grandparents. And why not? What Helen Keller is saying here is that she grew up. She no longer struggled against the world; instead she used what she had, and found peace and effectiveness. Choose a handicap in your practice and experiment with embracing it as Helen Keller embraced her own. Experience all of it—the resistance, the fear, the pain, and the possibility of growth. Experiment with being grateful for your handicaps.

DAY 152

There is no higher religion than human service.
To work for the common good is the greatest creed.

Albert Schweitzer

A while ago, I began dedicating my practice to the end of suffering. I had read in one of the Dalai Lama's books that he had taken a vow to end the suffering of all beings. This seemed like a great vow. For a time, I simply lamented not being a Tibetan monk. Then I began to consider ways in which I could make that vow my own. In many respects, it is a vow I had already taken, as a part of a twelve-step program. My life was already dedicated to service, which is twelve-step shorthand for alleviating suffering in others. But I wanted something more formal, a ritual way to extend my love even to those I will never see. All of my practices—my meditation practice, asana, *pranayama,* teaching, writing, twelve-step work—are meant to end my suffering. But there is more to it than that. I am a drop in the ocean, and as the content of my drop changes, the ocean changes, and as the ocean changes, I change. Dedicating my practice to the end of suffering connects to the underlying reality of the work that I do on myself. It connects me to the fact that there is no separation between me and all living beings. As I extend love to myself, in the form of my practice, I am extending love to all beings.

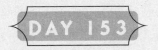

DAY 153

You can make more friends in two months by becoming interested in other people than you can in two years trying to get other people interested in you.

Dale Carnegie

No one told me this. I blundered around trying to be cool and interesting until the age of thirty. At thirty, I began working as an addictions counselor. In this line of work, being interested in other people is your full-time job. You are not trying to get sober; they are. So they become the only game in town. Your accomplishments, what you did on the weekend, how you feel about your parents or your job—none of that is of any importance in the central drama, which is whether or not your client will get sober. I learned an entirely new set of skills. Up until that time, I had devoted myself to being impressive. Now, suddenly, I was developing an interview style. I had a new aptitude for asking questions that you would want to answer. Within a few years, my life had transformed. I had developed the ability to form a community. I could chat with almost anyone, and feel nourished doing so. I had always had the ability; it had just never been tapped. I had been too busy being interesting.

Do not second-guess yourself on the mat, or underrate the power of asana. The fact that I had spent the first thirty years of my life trapped in a self-defeating behavior in no way indicated that I would, or should, spend the next thirty years in the same fashion. Whatever you were doing with your body before you came to the mat is in the past. You are in the right place at the right time, and the sky is the limit.

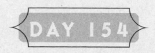

DAY 154

The human individual is equipped to learn and go on learning prodigiously from birth to death, and this is precisely what sets him or her apart from all other known forms of life. Man has at various times been defined as a building animal, a working animal, and a fighting animal, but all of these definitions are incomplete and finally false. Man is a learning animal, and the essence of the species is encoded in that simple term.

George Leonard

Practicing the asana, we reacquaint ourselves with this truth about ourselves on a daily basis. As a teacher I have developed a degree of mastery over a specific form of yoga. I've logged thousands of hours going over essentially the same postures in the same order. I never tire of this because every day is different. In class I often say that we can never enter the same river twice, experience the same posture twice, or take the same breath twice. Even on my worst days, as I trudge through my practice, I experience new levels of suppleness, balance, focus, and strength. This newness is something I have never experienced before. I am inhabiting my body and my life in a whole new way. Part of my commitment to learning, however, is to leave my familiar pond and try new waters.

As I write this, I am living in a town where Iyengar is spoken. I am a power yogi, and power yogis embrace the dance of it all, while Iyengar yogis embrace the precision of it all. It is therefore particularly good for me to drop into an Iyengar class every now and then, and to see my asana practice in a new light. The importance of doing this does not change the fact that the transition is hard. I usually spend my first couple of Iyengar classes moving between judgment and self-pity. Eventually, though, the breakthrough happens. Suddenly I am enjoying myself. I am learning! We enjoy our practice because, as we flow through the postures each day, we are learning, we are growing. Showing up for something different, being willing to be a beginner again, is one of the ways we keep our practice alive. We are here to learn.

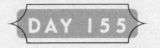

DAY 155

What I like about yoga is that it is not based on faith, it is based on experience. I know from experience that I carry stress in my body, and the postures are ways not only of releasing that stress, but confronting it, experiencing it, and understanding it. You have to learn to accept it, to live with it, and to let it go. You can apply that to a posture, or a fear, or whatever it is that is standing in the way of being at peace. The postures are one way of understanding these blockages, if you apply some wisdom to the practice, if you pay attention.

Clyde B., yoga student

Clyde and his wife, Rene, had been practicing yoga and meditation for some time before they began coming to my classes several years ago. They bring kindness, warmth, a smile, generosity, quiet strength, and maturity to the early-morning classes at the studio. Many young people attending college in Cambridge or experiencing their first years in the workforce begin their days in the presence of this outstanding couple. For many of us, they embody what we hope to become—strong and loving, wise and faithful. A devoted father, Clyde has been committed to social justice throughout his law career. So it is not surprising that he would focus on the asana as a practical, proven agent of change in our lives. On the mat we learn to confront, experience, understand, accept, live with, and let go of the difficulties of our lives. And in so doing we learn to live fully, as Clyde and Rene are doing one day at a time.

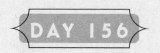

DAY 156

It don't make no difference to me, you believe what you want to believe, but you don't have to live like a refugee.

Tom Petty and the Heartbreakers

The Yoga Sutras are merely a reflection of what is. Generation after generation we are confronted by the same human predicament. The only thing that changes is how we write about it. Here, Tom Petty gives the second sutra on asana a contemporary spin. It seems that someone he loves believes she has to live like a refugee in the present, just because she has been "kicked around some" in the past. Clearly, her problem is the "natural tendencies" she developed as a result of her karma. The solution, of course, is a shift in perception. She can make a conscious choice to perceive something anew, to believe something else about herself. She must "meditate on the infinite" within herself.

How many of us join her every day by living like refugees in one way or another? The asana are our opportunity to deconstruct the refugee dynamic in our lives. On the mat, again and again, we encounter our limiting beliefs: we must do this, we can't do that. The sutras and Tom Petty are telling us that we can believe what we want to believe, but we certainly don't have to go on like this forever.

Identify one limiting belief that you act out on the mat every day. To begin, merely name it each time it comes up. For a while now, mine has been "toil." I choose to practice, then I lament it. Feeling sorry for myself, I "toil away." Each time my body language or thoughts turn to toil, I name it—without judgment or trying to change it. I merely make space for it in my awareness, allowing for the possibility that I am not a yoga refugee.

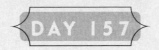

DAY 157

In the teaching-learning situation, each one learns
that giving and receiving are the same.

A Course in Miracles

In the Bhagavad Gita, yoga is called skillfulness in action. How does our work on the mat bring about skillfulness in our life off the mat? Let us begin with the asana as steady and sweet. What is happening when our postures are both steady and sweet? In headstand, the weight rests squarely on our shoulders, the legs come straight out of our hips, the balls of the feet press upward, the toes are awake. This is being steady, this is giving. In headstand we bring our attention to our center of gravity in the hips, and we achieve an exquisite balance so that the experience of the posture is effortless and focused. This is being sweet, this is receiving. We are not overly invested in either sweetness or steadiness, we are simply steady and sweet; giving and receiving occur simultaneously.

In our daily lives, we attend to our responsibilities, our duties, our spiritual practice, our worklife, our relationships. This is *dharma;* it is being steady, it is giving. In our daily lives, we are honest in our dealings with others, ensuring that we are fair and being fairly treated. We take action on our own behalf, seeing to it that we are living our dreams and being adequately compensated for the good that we do. This is *artha;* it is being sweet, it is receiving. We are not overly invested in either sweetness or steadiness, we are simply being steady and sweet; giving and receiving occur simultaneously. Thus it can be said that the asana teach skillfulness in life.

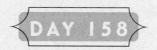

DAY 158

Whatever work we attempt cannot be perfectly done unless our minds are tranquil and calm.

Sri K. Pattabhi Jois

I had lunch the other day with a friend and fellow teacher, and we talked for a while about the fact that as our students become more dedicated, they also get to know more and more people in their classes. As a result, when we walk into class to teach, we find a veritable beehive of friendly chatter. The first ten minutes of class are devoted to rechanneling this energy. Whether you are practicing on your own or in class, take some time at the beginning of your practice to arrive. I begin my own practice with fifteen minutes of *pranayama,* reclining on my back with a bolster elevating my chest to assist the expansion of my lungs. This posture is physically and mentally relaxing, allowing me to become physically tranquil and calm.

The *pranayama* also calms and focuses my mind while it prepares my lungs for asana. Make a science of beginnings. Start to become conscious of the state of your mind as you assume the postures of your life.

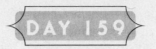

DAY 159

Begin your [asana practice] by sitting on the floor in any comfortable position. Feel the energy in the room. Observe the colors and shapes, and be aware of how you feel. Then close your eyes and breathe deeply, gently. Savor the air for a moment as you hold your breath, then release it slowly. Do this three times, reminding yourself that you are an integral part of the universe. Pay attention to your posture, the feeling-tone of you, and be relaxed and motionless. Then say a short prayer or invocation.

Erich Schiffmann

The habit of beginning your practice in an intentional way will permeate the rest of your life. For a few years, going to twelve-step meetings was my primary spiritual practice. Whenever I sat down at a meeting I would silently say, "Thank you for bringing me here." This has become a habit. Now, whenever I am at the start of something, I pause for a moment to say either, "Thy will be done," or, "Thank you for bringing me here." There is a pause in my beginnings, during which I align with the divine. And each time, I am reminded of the thousands of other times I have paused before, of the now countless moments of deep connection, of their beauty, and of my place in the universe.

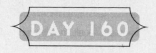

Only through skill does balance come.

Donna Farhi

Firm and relaxed, steady and sweet, effortless and focused—where do these words lead? In daily life, we're bombarded by sensation: sights, sounds, smells, physical sensations, fantasies and memories, hopes and dreams, fears and realities, duties and responsibilities, everything from the fact of our mortality to the need to buy some more toilet paper. This bombardment overstimulates us and we become reactive. Saturated by experience, we lose sight of who we are. We react in the moment, out of the tangle of past experiences. So, a red light is not just a red light, it is all of the times I have been late, all of the times I haven't been late, what the army taught me about being on time, what I imagine others will think of me for being late . . . Somewhere underneath all this there might even lurk the fact that I don't want to go wherever it is I am going at the moment, so I am dragging my feet. All of this and a whole lot more inform my reaction to the stoplight. In the chaos of overstimulated reactivity, clear seeing becomes an impossibility, skillfulness in action irrelevant. My thoughts, my words, and my deeds don't add up; I am living in illusion.

Yoga opposes this condition with practices aimed at quieting the mind, the body, and the spirit. On the mat, we have a microcosm of our lives. Bombarded with sensation, we can become overwhelmed and reactive, or we can begin to acquire skill in the art of life. Where do we begin? I suppose we could start with the words "firm and relaxed," "steady and sweet," "effortless and focused," and see what happens.

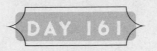

You, just as you are, and your life here, right now, are all there is
and all you need to know. You don't have to do anything special.
Mostly, you have to be open to meeting face to face, and even
dancing with, the truth that pertains to your life right now. You
have to find a way to collect your fractured pieces, examine
them, and then accept them as part of who you are. Spiritual
practice is about transformation, but it's also, and more
importantly, about working with what is.

Angel Kyodo Williams

I came to the practice of asana with a curvature in my spine. Thousands of
hours of my life have been devoted to struggling with the effects of this. On
the mat, my lower back became a battleground. I fought and lost, fought
and lost. My efforts to heal myself often ended in debilitating back spasms.
Over time, though, I began to respect my back. I marveled at its ability to
bend backward and forward, to recover from tremendously painful injuries.
Eventually I started to befriend my back, and even to see it as something to
be admired. I began focusing on what it could do. As this attitude developed, the need to change my back, to fight my reality, lessened and gradually disappeared. The curvature in my back is gone, and I can't remember
exactly when it went away, because when it did, I no longer cared.

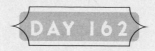
You have to keep showing up, being open, and doing the work. The journey into the self is not a group experience. It's solitary work. But so many of us are afraid of being alone. So you need to experiment. . . . The whole process of following these spiritual instructions has a lot to do with conquering our fear.

Beryl Bender Birch

One of the questions I return to regularly is, "What am I afraid of?" Of course, I see many people in class who are afraid of falling out of headstand or pitching forward onto their faces in crow pose. But this isn't exactly what I mean. Every few months, I seem to see anew that there are many aspects of my practice either that are stuck or that I approach in a manner that ensures that I will only scratch the surface. Recently I caught myself saying in a class in which I was a student, "I never do it that way, and I have been successful." In that moment, I brought myself up short and asked, "Have I?" Have I truly lived up to my potential? The answer was no. In fact, one of the reasons I'm such a devoted practitioner is that I know I have not lived up to my potential. In that moment, I took one more small step on the solitary journey into myself. I caught myself in one of the habitual attitudes that have blocked me from new ways of experiencing myself and my potential. What am I afraid of? What are you afraid of?

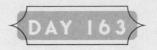

A S A N A

I started yoga because I was looking for something holistic. I had gone to a body worker who told me that I wasn't breathing enough, that I wasn't breathing deeply enough, and that was a real metaphor for where I was in my life at the time. I felt as though I was just going through the motions of living and not really admitting it.

Gil C., yoga student

Gil describes the condition many of us are in when we first come to yoga, whether we are aware of it or not. We have retreated from many aspects of ourselves, and therefore many areas of our lives are literally unknown to us, unexamined and unlived in. In yoga classes, this situation is not subtle. New students, for example, do not inhabit their hands. In postures in which their arms are extended, their hands stick out of their arms in limp, random, lifeless arrangements. Most of us come to yoga having retreated from our hands, our feet, our hips, our hearts and lungs, our entire bodies. We have become terrified of our own reality, the great unknown. The asana are a series of controlled experiments in reinhabiting our bodies. One of the words for body that I like best is the Greek word *soma,* which means the home of the spirit. Somewhere along the line, our bodies have fallen asleep, our *soma*s are dusty and grown over with vines. The asana are like the prince who comes to awaken the sleeping princess, breathing life back into lifeless limbs.

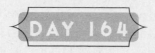

> However often the restless mind may break loose and wander,
> he should rein it in and constantly bring it back to the self.
>
> Bhagavad Gita

The first time I taught meditation, the class sold out for the season. On the first night all went well. We practiced asana, then *pranayama,* then sat in stillness. Everyone in the class was new to meditation, but they had all heard good things about it and spirits were high. At the beginning of the second class, I addressed what the Buddhists call the Noble Failure. The Noble Failure is the truth we learn when we first begin to meditate or practice asana, which is that we cannot control our minds. We bring our minds to one point, then they drift off somewhere else, and we must start all over again. This encounter with our restless minds, and our inability to do anything about them, is called the Noble Failure. The Noble Failure is why we need to practice in the first place. I went on to play a tape in which a meditation teacher describes meditation as being similar to being locked in a closet with a maniac. No one laughed. And that was the beginning of my own less-than-noble failure as a meditation teacher. By the next week, a third of the class had bailed. "No, we don't need our money back," was the message, "just get us the hell out of here." By the end of the eight-week session, only a third of the students were left.

There is something to be said for skillful instruction, but it remains a daunting proposition to find out just how out of control our minds really are. The only option we have is to patiently train our minds, the way we would train a dog or a child. The asana give us a fairly gentle circumstance in which to train our minds to stay in the present. There is a lot to do—we have to breathe, we have to know what's going on with our feet, our hips, our knees, our shoulders, our spines, our gaze, our effort, our effortlessness. When we are busy with all of this, it is usually immediately apparent when our minds wander off, and it does not take a great deal of self-control to bring them back to the matter at hand. Nevertheless, this work is excellent training for the mind. Begin to watch this same dynamic off the mat, and see if you are not improving. Observe your conversations, and see if your asana practice hasn't made you a better listener.

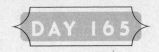

Without concern for results, perform the necessary action; surrendering all attachments, accomplish life's highest good.

Bhagavad Gita

Once we are under way, how do we proceed? Consider the moments when you were most effective in your life—that night when you could have danced forever, that test you aced, the job you finished so well. By and large, when we look back on our best efforts we realize that they occur in moments of nonattachment to results. We are doing the thing because we love the thing itself. We are in the moment without thought of the next moment. Unfortunately, we can remember these moments because they tend to be so extraordinary, so rare in our lives. For most of us, acting out of desire or aversion is the ordinary. Life is a struggle—to gain something or to avoid something. In order for this not to be so, we have to take a few steps back and answer a couple of questions—first, "What am I?" and second, "What am I not?"

Yoga suggests that you are divine consciousness on a divine mission to realize the truth about yourself. Do you believe this? Do you believe this to be true of all beings? Could you try it on at the beginning of your next practice? Begin to ask yourself, "What am I?" and, "What am I not?" when you feel desire or aversion coming up, whether on or off the mat. See if letting go begins to make more sense when you are not defined by the results of your actions. Imagine that your life is meant to be a dance in which you are held in the embrace of all living beings.

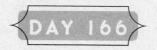

DAY 166

If a man has done his best, what else is there?

George S. Patton Jr.

Because of my asana practice, I experience a deeper level of dignity in my life. Over and over again, I show up on my mat just not in the mood. Something has not gone my way, or I may simply be tired. In any case, my heart is not in it. But I start anyway. At these times, I appreciate the fact that I start with fifteen minutes of reclining *pranayama,* because I can fling my weary body down and lie flat on my back, arms outstretched. I stay with the breath, move through the exercise, connect to the expansiveness in my chest. I perform one sun salutation, and then I say the ancient mantra "om" three times. "Om" is the name, the sound, and the vibration of divinity. I experience the name, sound, and vibration of God in every cell in my body. I "om" my powerlessness, I "om" my gratitude, I "om" to end the suffering of all beings. Then I begin. Some days it turns around and I get a surge of energy; some days it doesn't. It doesn't really matter. If I complete my practice, which is most days, I can step back and let go. I have done my best. What else is there?

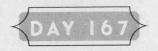

It is easier to act yourself way into a better way of feeling,
than to feel yourself into a better way of action.

O. H. Mowrer

In twelve-step programs, people going through a difficult time in their lives will often say they are "staying close to the program." Staying close to the program means staying close to your supports, your friends and mentors, and using your practices. The counsel to "stay close to the program" recognizes our tendency to retreat from spiritual practice in times of acute stress. In my own asana practice, "staying close to the program" means building time for practice into a difficult week or a challenging day. It also means taking right action when I am not at all in the mood.

Early on the morning of September 11, my wife and I narrowly missed getting on the wrong plane. We ended up stranded in a Miami hotel for four days, watching CNN and eating ice cream. My first practice after this emotionally wrenching time was, in all honesty, unpleasant. I had not been "staying close to the program" as far as asana goes and my diet had been poor. As I trudged my way through my practice, I coached myself: "This is a system for mental, physical, and spiritual health and you badly need all three right now, so use the system. You don't have to excel, you don't have to worry about the implications of not excelling, you just need to use the system." It worked beautifully. Oftentimes when we need yoga the most, we want it the least.

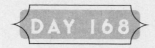

DAY 168

You are the bows from which your children as living arrows are
sent forth. The archer sees the mark upon the path of the
infinite, and He bends you with His might that His arrows may
go swift and far. Let your bending in the archer's hand be for
gladness; for even as He loves the arrow that flies, so He loves
also the bow that is stable.

Kahlil Gibran

Some of us have children now, some of us will have children some day, and
some of us will never have children. The practice of yoga encourages the
birth of a different kind of children, the children of our art. These children
are the works of art and selfless service that we bring into the world. They
are the love we share with the world that is uniquely ours. As practitioners
of yoga, we come to see that no moment, no act, is ordinary—they are all
our children. The asana make us a stable bow from which these children can
fly. "Let your bending in the archer's hand be for gladness."

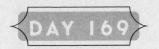

A S A N A

Surrender is not achieved until you surrender completely
to your beloved. To accomplish this you must relinquish
everything that deprives you of love and nurture everything
that comes from love.

Deepak Chopra

We are children of the light, born in darkness. Most of us like what we know, and what we know is darkness. The extent to which this is true is easily ascertained by making your asana practice a meditation.

Try this: At the beginning of your next practice, tell yourself, "I will keep my mind in the now. I will devote my attention solely to the posture I am in right now." Then watch as your mind refuses to cooperate. Stay with it and, as you do so, lighten up. Let go of the frustration and the judgment, and work with your unruly mind as you would with a child or a puppy. It is very important that you come to know this unruliness in yourself and that you be willing to embrace it, not judge it.

It is only with an adequate understanding of our untamed mind that we can begin to understand the nature of our suffering, the meaning of the word surrender, and the point of spiritual practice. This understanding is our first step into the light.

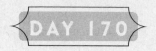

The conjunction of the seer with the seen is for the seer to discover his own true nature.

Yoga Sutras

This is good news. We've heard the bad news: we don't know who we are, which gives us an exaggerated sense of I-ness and pride, which in turn tethers us to an endless round of fear and desire. And if that's not bad enough, we're not even supposed to be afraid of death. So, what's the good news?

The good news is that all of this, every last aspect of this experience called life, has only one purpose: our spiritual growth. The intersection of the spiritual with the physical, energy with matter, life with the lifeless, all has evolution as its aim. It is all about evolution, and we are invited to the party. That is, if we choose to go.

Krishnamurti said that we do not learn from experience; rather, we learn from the experiences we choose to learn from. It's all about evolution—if we are willing to see it that way. We have free will. The eight-limb path's solutions to life's difficulties offer us a means for making systematic our choice to learn from experience. Yoga is a means for cultivating personal responsibility for our own growth. The practices, the *yamas,* the *niyamas,* asana, *pranayama,* and meditation are merely invitations to partake more fully, more completely, in the divine dance.

We have a sense of the problem, and if you are at all like me, you have more than a sense that you have lived it. Now, let's embrace the solution. Start where you are. Begin to see your entire life as your spiritual practice. Whether it is thanking the person who opens the door for you, giving a good tip to your waiter, or the hours you spending sweating on your mat, embrace your place in the moment with all your heart.

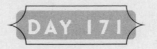

*Any fact facing us is not as important as our attitude toward it,
for that determines our success or failure.*

Norman Vincent Peale

The asana require us to take responsibility for our physical as well as our mental attitude. Good attitude, good results; bad attitude, bad results. Not long ago I watched a video in which six of the most accomplished yogis in the United States practice with their teacher. Their body language is eloquent with mastery. The next day, inspired by their example, I tried practicing using the same body language. My body was saying, "And now, Rolf, the world's greatest yogi, will flow seamlessly from one posture to the next." What I found was that my practice improved dramatically. I *was* flowing seamlessly from posture to posture. The body language of mastery is the body language of balance, confidence and grace, precision and simplicity. It is the body language of a positive attitude. Practicing the asana, we have the opportunity to bring our internal and external attitudes into alignment.

DAY 172

There is no such thing as my body or your body except in words.
Of the one huge mass of matter, one point is called a moon,
another a sun, another a man, another the earth, another a
plant, another a mineral.

Swami Vivekananda

When I attempt a posture that's new for me, or difficult, there is usually a sense of separation. I can't help but think of all those people, through the centuries, who were able to do this posture. Oftentimes I look around and see that those close to me can do it, my wife can do it, sometimes even my dog can do it—but I cannot. Isolated, alone on my island of no-can-do, I make halfhearted attempts at performing a posture I know is beyond my abilities. Then one day, because I practice regularly, I am temporarily over my self-pity. I come to the same posture with a different attitude. I call to mind an image of the posture done correctly. I imagine that within me is the ability to perform this posture effortlessly. I move toward the posture calmly, deliberately, without fear or desire, only interest and pleasure. On this day I am able either to perform the posture or at least to begin to understand it. This understanding leaves an imprint on my central nervous system and in my cells that I will be able to return to the next day. I experience a connection to the posture by which I am forever changed.

Caught in the grip of ego, or *asmita,* the exaggerated sense of I-ness, we find that many postures are beyond us. The asana require us to get over our sense of separateness. They bring us home to the plain truth that we are not separate. On the contrary, we each hold within us the entire experience of the universe, as surely as the universe contains us. It is because of this that we are able to effortlessly perform the asana. Observe the experience of inability and the experience of ability in your practice.

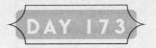

The word "innocence" comes from Latin and means "not harmful." This is also the first concept in the ancient yoga texts: *ahimsa,* or nonviolence, nonharmfulness. True artists, as well as true yogis, have their being in this innocence and joyfulness, which comes from standing alone in the world, looking at it with eyes which are empty of rules and measures, and reflecting this innocence and joy, in body, mind, and emotions. This is the stamp of really great artists. And in the ultimate analysis, each one of us is an artist.

Dona Hollemann

When I'm in the midst of my asana practice, the Yoga Sutras serve both as an outline for my experience and as my personal trainer. In the kaleidoscope of sensations that is my experience of practice, the key words of the sutras on asana serve as an anchor. "Firm and relaxed," "steady and sweet," "effortless and focused," "letting go of past conditioning and meditating on the infinite"—these words are the container. What is the experience?

Astanga yoga teacher Beryl Bender Birch uses the word "unspeakable" to describe the experience of yoga practice. As she points out, one person cannot describe the experience of hearing a piece of music to another—we must hear it for ourselves. Much of the rest of this section will address the unspeakable. We will revisit the *yamas* and *niyamas* in the context of our daily asana practice, and we will use the words of students and teachers to infuse and inform our own experience of the unspeakable with the collective wisdom of brothers and sisters who are on this path with us. Together, we will stand alone and look upon the world with eyes empty of rules and measures, as artists whose lives are our art.

DAY 174

I was looking for something to help me feel stronger. I also needed to feel more grounded or rooted in my body. When I started practicing yoga, I felt my spine and the life of my spine. The impact of building core strength has been freeing in so many ways. Yoga has helped connect me to the fact that we really are bodies.

After a month my body just changed. I feel a much stronger connection to my hands and feet, the top of my head and spine. I feel much more alive. Yoga has helped me understand that I can't keep denying that I have a body. I have to deal with my physicality. I am beginning to see that being a physical being is a path, not a limitation.

Dave E., yoga student

I met Dave when we were both in school to become social workers. The program was intense and Dave and I had to get up very early in order to practice. I would practice yoga and he would practice tai chi. Our paths continued to cross after we left school and eventually he began coming to my studio. An aspect of his practice is service to the community. Dave and his dad, Dave Senior, have put in hundreds of hours painting and improving the studio. Thousands of people have benefited from the work of the two Daves, without ever knowing it.

Dave's observations go right to the heart of an important aspect of the genius of the asana. We are embodied. Many spiritual paths sidestep this truth. The asana confronts it head-on. Our spiritual exploration of this life begins with our bodies. We start right where we are. We end our wars with our bodies, and we begin the practice of love.

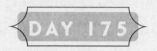

DAY 175

Our aim must never be to defeat or humiliate the white man
but to win his friendship and understanding.

Martin Luther King Jr.

Ahimsa, or nonviolence, is the core teaching of yoga. The easiest way to stay on track in your asana practice is to remember this. In my own practice, the importance of nonviolence on the mat has taken hold slowly, over the course of a number of years. The first physical disciplines I practiced were aimed at defeating and humiliating my opponents in sports. Of course, my body often ended up on the wrong side of the battle. It would frequently send me impertinent memos concerning proper nutrition and rest. Smoking was another bone of contention, not to mention the vats of alcohol I asked it to contend with. On the whole, my body cooperated as best it could. But paired with a psyche at war with reality, my body never lived up to its potential.

The shift has been slow but wondrous, and there have been too many layers of growth and transformation to mention them all. Suffice it to say that as we begin to honor and care for our bodies, our entire lives begin to change. The sensitivity necessary for us to become conscious of all the ways we act against our own bodies will ultimately teach us to avoid pitfalls in our everyday lives as well. As we explore our relationships with our bodies, we see the imprint of all our other relationships. We begin to see the true nature of our beliefs concerning politics, gender, sex, money, power, the whole enchilada. On the mat we venture out into the wilderness of our karma. The practice of *ahimsa* is crucial on this journey. We must not stand in judgment of ourselves. Our aim must never be to defeat or humiliate, but to befriend and understand.

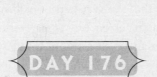

DAY 176

Yet this we ask of you ere you leave us,
that you speak to us and give us of your truth.

Kahlil Gibran

The second value in yoga is honesty, or *satya*. On the mat, this *yama* translates as humility. Humility is often confused with humiliation—but humility does not cause humiliation, it prevents it. Humility is not being humble, it is being honest. It is being right sized. There is no love for this virtue in our culture. Our leaders hail us as the greatest superpower of all time, our heroes trumpet, "I'm on top of the world!" and new yoga students have disdain for the block and the strap (they're for sissies). I have had to stop using the word "advanced" in class to describe a posture, because if I do, everyone tries it. We have not been taught to be honest with ourselves or with others.

Honesty is actually the moment when life starts to get good. We let go, simultaneously, of the fear that has made us obscure our truth and the strain of presenting a false self to the world. Becoming right sized, for most of us, is a serious promotion. Under our delusions of grandeur lurks the certainty of mediocrity. Becoming right sized means letting go of the pretense that we are not God's children, that we are not born divine. The paradox is that even as we recognize our own divinity, we must also be willing to go back to square one. The asana present us with an inexhaustible supply of opportunities to go back to square one, to develop humility. If we are willing to do this, a beautiful thing happens—an authentic human being begins to emerge. As this being matures, we find that we do have something to say, something to share, and that the very acts of telling and sharing are healing for both the giver and the receiver. The asana embody this knowledge; they remind us, over and over again, that before we leave this short life, we must give of our truth.

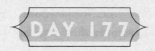

On my way back from my first class, I called my husband
and said, "I have just found what I've been looking for." I was
transformed almost immediately. Within a month I thought
completely differently—emotionally and spiritually. Yoga
dissipates fear. My fear had created illusions, and my illusions
had kept me a prisoner in a life that I was not happy with,
a life that was not me.
Before yoga, I had a nagging suspicion that something was off. I
had had a lot of success in sports and academics, but my success
had been an escape, a way to get approval, and this culture
really rewarded me. I was a huge success, but I was empty and
yearning inside.
Yoga breaks down the barriers to knowing your true self. Before
yoga, I would get sporadic glimpses of that self. But when I
didn't have sight of my soul, or true being, I was not existing on
all levels—physical, spiritual, emotional, mental. Yoga allows me
to balance all four levels. On the mat, I am faced with *me*—this
beautiful soul, with all of this clutter. Yoga clears the clutter.

Leigh H., yoga student

Leigh's observations capture the essence of *satya,* or truthfulness, on the
mat. As we grow in integrity on the mat, we grow in authenticity off the
mat. The attunement to the moment and to the real that is required by our
yoga practice does not leave us when we leave the mat. Rather, it brings our
lives into focus. From Leigh we get a sense of the holistic nature of the
growth that occurs both on the mat and off. We get a sense that a seed was
planted at her first class, and that it has flourished. Her progress has not been

without trials but her commitment to daily practice offsets the hardships she encounters. Through her practice, Leigh has found the means to give of her truth.

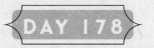

DAY 178

Take no thought, saying, What shall we eat? or, What shall we drink? or, Wherewithal shall we be clothed? For your heavenly Father knoweth that ye have need of all these things. But seek ye first the kingdom of God, and his righteousness: and all these things shall be added unto you.

Matthew 6:31–33

The third principle in yoga is *asteya,* or nonstealing. The simplest way to define nonstealing is acting in faith. And the simplest way to define stealing is faithlessness. Long before the actual act of stealing, we believe that we will not be taken care of; we lose faith in right action. On the mat we are given the opportunity to experience our fear of not being taken care of. It comes to us as a thousand concerns: "Am I doing it right?" "Am I doing it enough?" "Should I do more?" "Should I do less?" If we are in the posture, the answers to these questions will come to us—but we cannot truly be in the posture and be asking these questions at the same time. It is that simple. Our faithlessness blocks our growth. Our faithlessness steals the moment away, from ourselves and from the universe. Let go into right action, and let that be enough. Be in the posture you are in right now, and let the rest of it sort itself out on its own.

> While washing the dishes one should only be washing the
> dishes, which means that while washing the dishes one should
> be completely aware of the fact that one is washing the dishes.
> At first glance, that might seem silly: Why put so much stress
> on a simple thing? But that's the point. The fact that I am
> standing there washing these bowls is a wondrous reality. I'm
> being completely myself, following my breath, conscious of my
> presence, and conscious of my thoughts and actions. There is no
> way I can be tossed around mindlessly like a bottle slapped here
> and there on the waves.
>
> Thich Nhat Hanh

I was being tossed around mindlessly like a bottle on the waves myself when I dashed into a store and bought Thich Nhat Hanh's book for a friend who had been taking care of my dog. I paged through it quickly, to make sure she would find it helpful, and this paragraph jumped out at me. I was actually in a great deal of pain, agonizing over a rather serious business decision. Because of this pressing situation, I had been unable to be truly present for anything for days. The experience of not being present is agitation. You may be distracted by a good thing or a bad thing, but agitation is draining in either case.

My spiritual batteries were empty—so empty, in fact, that I could not imagine how to fill them. After buying the book, I (rather desperately) began paying attention to what I was doing. Not to what I might be doing in the future, but to what I was doing right now. The relief I felt was remarkable. I became a sane adult again. How to proceed in the business matter suddenly seemed less important; it was no big deal, because I was no longer attached to the outcome. My daily routine and my asana practice became nourishing again, for I was no longer stealing those moments away from myself.

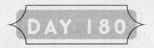

DAY 180

Friends brought me to my first yoga class, but told me nothing. I didn't even know there were poses! I didn't really like it, but for some reason I found myself going back two days later, and then again, two days after that. I felt as if I had to go. At first I didn't even want to buy a mat. I didn't think I really wanted to commit to it at that level.
Yoga was physical for me at first, but it is not that physical now. It taught me that I need to continue to work on myself. I thought it would be too selfish to concentrate on myself, because my purpose in life is to give. But with yoga practice new things come up all the time. I have a new awareness. I have had to look at my own honesty quite a bit. At a teacher training, two friends confronted me about the fact that I have always liked to put things in a "nice way"—not that I lie, but I don't always face things honestly. This used to affect me in my relationships. Now I ask myself, "Am I being honest with myself here? How do I really feel?" I have become more thoughtful, and I try to find the balance, which is yoga.

Caroline B., yoga student

Caroline, an ophthalmologist, spends a good deal of time overseas, donating her services to those in need. As she describes her growing commitment to her practice, we see how she is removing the borders in her own consciousness. We are able to observe how the *yamas,* the *niyamas,* and the asana occur simultaneously. The asana taught Caroline about the *yamas* of balance and honesty and the *niyamas* of self-study and commitment to practice. Overarching all of this is a gradual surrender. Caroline's story is like so many of ours. We come to the mat with no idea of what we are getting into or why. Slowly we begin to grow in awareness, and we find, looking back, that our arrival on the mat was right on time. And to the extent that we are willing to give of ourselves to this process, we receive the benefits of it.

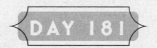

Force is all conquering but its victories are short lived.

Abraham Lincoln

The fourth *yama* is *brahmacarya,* or moderation. When it comes to applying this *yama* on the mat, Abraham Lincoln pretty much says it all. We have to be willing to give time. Attempting to cram ten years' worth of asana practice into a couple of years won't work. *Brahmacarya* on the mat is about finding a practice that is sustainable. It is also about finding a practice that supports your life off the mat. Stephen King advises writers not to place their desks in the middle of a room but to the side, as a reminder that writing should not be at the center of one's life. He goes on to remind us that life should be at the center of one's life. This is *brahmacarya* on the mat, steady and sweet, firm and relaxed, focused and effortless.

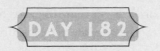

ASANA

We shape the clay into a pot, but it is the emptiness inside
that holds whatever we want.

Lao-Tzu

Aparigraha, or nonhoarding, is the art of appreciating emptiness in one's life, but before we can learn to appreciate emptiness, we must first learn to let go. On the mat we practice *aparigraha* by letting go of our expectations and letting go of the concerns of the day. I recently caught myself comparing a class I was taking to another class that I had found more fulfilling. I paused then and questioned my belief that the other class had somehow been more satisfying. I realized that the class I had found more fulfilling was one in which I had surrendered more deeply, one in which I had given a big sigh, let go of my day, and relaxed into the moment—with no thought of how it should be, no repeated clock checks, just childlike compliance and present-moment awareness. I had allowed that class to be fulfilling simply by letting go into it. I had to admit now that I was making a choice not to be fulfilled by the class I was in, that I was so full of my own expectations that I could not receive from the class I was taking. *Aparigraha* reminds us to always let go and never hold on. This letting go is the cultivation of emptiness in our lives. Into this emptiness, grace will come.

About a year and a half ago I left Colorado, where I
had been living for many years, on the tail end of a bad
relationship. I needed distance. . . . I had thrown myself
into this relationship, and I had left myself out, and now I
felt utterly empty. I was aware that I was searching for
something, and after I regained some of my strength, I
began reaching out to things I'd had an interest in but had
never done. After my first yoga class I was floored. For the
first time in a long while, I sensed that everything was going
to be OK, that things would get better if I continued to
stay focused on this, on me. At the time, I was hurt and
self-conscious about where I was at. People would ask
what I did or where I was going, and I was unemployed,
with no answers. At the studio, I didn't have to know. I
was healing financially and emotionally, and class was a
sanctuary. I was learning how to handle the hurt and the
anger because I was focused on me. In class I didn't need
an answer for why things happened; I could just let go. At
the studio I finally felt as if I fit in.
I have been physical, but also very competitive, all my life.
Yoga was the one area in my life where I didn't compete.
I've settled into being a student. I am willing to learn, but
it's not about getting better, or better than the person
next to me. Now I admire the other students for their
dedication. Yoga has cleared my mind, and my decision
making is better. I'm enjoying my life right now and am
thankful that the relationship didn't work out, and that

my path brought me here. I am content with who I am, and
the happiness is exploding inside me.

Laura S., yoga student

Laura is emptying her cup, and grace is pouring in.

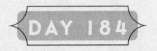

DAY 184

These forms are not the means for obtaining
the right state of mind. To take this posture is itself
to have the right state of mind.

Suzuki Roshi

As the students' stories unfold we see again and again that the asana bring with them a new awareness, a shift in focus. Our old ways of thinking dictated our previous physicality, and as we experience a new physicality, we experience new ways of thinking. To truly understand this is to catch a glimpse of interconnectedness. The central nervous system informs the cells, and the cells inform the central nervous system. Information flows back and forth like the tide. There is no hierarchy, no separation, no moment when the man in the white coat and the letters next to his name says, "This is true, this is not true." There is only the real—your truth, perceived in the moment, heard in your soul. The asana are a dance of the real, a dance with our truth. Over time this dance changes the way we see the world. What more fundamental change is there?

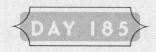

For those who are completely attached to enjoyment and power, with the mind carried away by it, their wisdom, which is the essence of will, is not settled in samadhi.

Bhagavad Gita

In this translation, *samadhi* means clear seeing. Attachment clouds our judgment, but letting go of our attachment is an enormous challenge to those of us who wish to use the asana as a means for spiritual transformation. We can practice yoga simply as a means for physical well-being. If, however, we choose to make the asana an integral aspect of our spiritual path, the stakes become very high. As we invest more of ourselves in our practice, the desire for certainty grows. We wish to enjoy the assurance that we have found the one true way. But such certainty cannot be found outside ourselves, and we are always changing. If we are not steadfastly prepared to let go of yesterday's truths, we fall prey to the fundamentalism found in any of the major religions; we begin to believe that this way is good, that way is bad; this yoga is right, and that yoga is wrong. Clear seeing must be more important to us than the comfort of certainty, the power of feeling that we know. The letting go on the mat must be absolute. We must be beyond all opposites, anchored in the real, empty and clear.

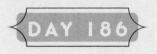

And how shall you rise beyond your days and nights unless you
break the chains which you have fastened around your noon
hour? In truth that which you call freedom is the strongest
of these chains, though its links glitter in the sun and
dazzle your eyes.

Kahlil Gibran

The first *niyama* is *sauca,* or purity. *Sauca* on the mat is the work that we do
to prepare our bodies and our minds to realize the opportunity of asana. For
me, it primarily concerns diet, rest, meditation, and avoidance of overwork
and overtraining. The result of purity on the mat is a pliant, strong, sensitive, balanced body, a focused mind, and a carefree spirit. We achieve these
things through the voluntary surrender of certain freedoms.

If I am unwilling to give up a few of my rights—my right to potato
chips and cream cheese brownies, for example, or my right to the money I
can earn by overworking, or my freedom to stay up until three to finish a
good book—then I will not realize my full potential on the mat. It's that
simple. Fortunately, the asana detoxify us, so that our desire for many of the
things we must give up lessens and disappears over time. Still, we are human,
and our distractions and appetites are part of who we are—certainly
enough so for *sauca* to continue to be a major player on the mat. Each of us
must determine for ourselves what *sauca* on the mat means to us. The asana
give us excellent feedback. When I am eating the wrong foods, my practice
is directly affected; it feels as if someone has poured sand in my gas tank. I
lose strength, focus, and sensitivity. Slogging through a practice when I'm
weakened by poor nutrition, I am forced to reconsider my definition of
freedom. *Sauca,* the first *niyama,* reminds us to apply the *yamas* on the mat.

⟨ DAY 187 ⟩

Both yoga and art aim at the same thing, that is, to re-establish
our personal connection with the world around us according to
our own inner creativity. To render body and mind a conduit
through which the creative energy can flow freely, unimpeded
by outer restrictions, in the trust that this energy, being a part
of the universal energy, is ultimately "pure" and joyful.

Dona Hollemann

This is the work of *sauca,* "to render body and mind a conduit through which the creative energy can flow freely." It is a noble endeavor. The asana do much of the work for us. They cleanse the organs, the central nervous system, the respiratory system, and the mind, while strengthening the muscular-skeletal system. Much can be accomplished through the asana, but not all. For each of us, *sauca* is a journey of discovery. What works for you? Dairy, no dairy; meat, no meat; lots of sunshine, very little sun; lots of stimulation, or quiet solitude; long ambles, or power walks. We each find our own way to health and balance. Once again, we are on the path that leads to the truth, and the means for determining the truth is our own individual experience. What practices render you a conduit through which the creative energy can flow freely?

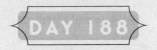

I have had fibrocystic breast disease. Within the first month of yoga, the disease—and all of the painful symptoms—went away completely. Emotionally, I felt as if I had let go of something, and then I realized that my illness was completely gone. Yoga makes me feel more like taking care of myself, so I am more conscious of what I put into my body, and I am more present, more aware of how things are affecting me. I feel more committed to taking care of myself.

Amy L., yoga student

To practice the asana under adequate instruction is to practice the *yamas* and *niyamas.* Amy describes how her practice facilitated an immediate and profound experience of *sauca,* or purity. Her story depicts a deep cleansing of her body and emotions, which is supported by a shift in her relationship to herself. She is experiencing *sauca* in the fullest sense of the word, and she achieved this by showing up on her mat.

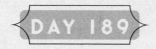

DAY 189

True ambition is the desire to live usefully and walk humbly
under the grace of God.

Bill Wilson

The second *niyama* is *santosa,* or contentment. On the mat, *santosa* is the experience of peace. It is that moment when we are no longer at war with ourselves but are content with what is, right now. Laura S. described her experience of *santosa* when she said, "Yoga was the one area in my life where I didn't compete. I've settled into being a student. I am willing to learn, but it's not about getting better, or better than the person next to me. Now I admire the other students for their dedication." These are the words of someone in harmony with her surroundings. Many students describe coming to yoga with vague feelings of discontent and moving toward a deepening experience of peace and happiness, a growing sense that, as Laura said, "everything was going to be OK." The asana give us this, but we must also be willing to meet them halfway. Bill Wilson also writes, "All by himself, and in the light of his own circumstances, he needs to develop the quality of willingness." In other words, we must be willing to be helped. We find contentment on our mats when we are finally willing to let go of the false pretenses that block contentment, when we acquire true ambition.

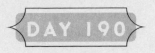

I have two daughters, and when they went off to college I began
to realize that they had given me my purpose in life, my purpose
beyond myself. This change, and reaching the midpoint in my
life, set me thinking. It was clear to me that I was hungry
spiritually. Middle age is the time when you realize that you are
going to die. Yoga has helped me to live through that realization, and to figure out what I'm going to do about it. A key
question for me has been, "How do I commit?" The first year
and a half of yoga was really hard, emotionally and physically,
and I wanted to quit. There were so many painful things, I
sometimes didn't know how I would get through class, but I
stayed with it. I think some of what I was learning by sticking
with yoga was also helping me to learn how to stick with my
partner. I worked on not leaving when the going gets tough.
And practicing this, living it, has helped me a lot with my
partner and at my new job. Yoga helps me to focus on the task
at hand, do it well, and not worry about what is going to
happen next.

Martha M., yoga student

Martha talks about the complexity beneath a simple concept. Contentment
in and of itself is not complex. Contentment is simply reverence for the
grace that is already present in our lives. On the mat, anchored in the real,
we encounter another aspect of *santosa*. Most of us arrive with a powerful
discontent practice already in place. To make matters worse, we live in an
ever-changing world that seems dedicated to providing us with opportunities for discontent. Martha discovered that the distance between discontent

and contentment is bridged by the willingness to be honest and to work hard. For Martha, the work has been to stay in one place and to let go of the results. She has had to learn to allow her truth to be enough, and by doing so she has opened the door to *santosa,* inviting contentment to become an aspect of her everyday life.

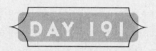

DAY 191

The human heart yearns for the beautiful in all ranks of life.

Harriet Beecher Stowe

The next *niyama* we encounter on the mat is *tapas,* literally translated as "heat," or burning zeal in practice. The word that most of us use to describe this energy is "dedication." This is not the dedication of steely self-control, it's the dedication of the human heart that yearns for beauty. It is our own capacity for love that underlies our ability to practice with burning zeal, year after year. Again and again students say they came to yoga to work on their flexibility, or to tone their abs, buns, and thighs, but that something else has kept them coming back. Something else has blossomed in their hearts. Yoga opens the door to the life that we have yearned to live. It is this yearning, this gladness, that carries us back onto our mats day after day. *Tapas* is our opportunity to witness the power of love in our everyday lives. As you approach your next practice, note the force that brings you to the mat. See if you can discern, under the clamor of desire and aversion, the still, pure voice that yearns for beauty.

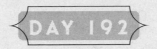

ASANA

> I came to yoga for the cross-training benefits, but after a while
> a few classes turned into more. I didn't see the effects right
> away, but then, all of a sudden, I was doing things that I could
> never do before. I am much more in tune with my body. Yoga
> makes me feel better mentally. I feel calmer and I can really let
> things go. Now I'm finding that I want more. I'm taking every
> move deeper, I'm wanting to hold the postures more deeply, and
> I want to understand more about yoga.
>
> Vicki E., yoga student

The asana awaken a momentum in our lives, and that momentum is *tapas*. Vicki's experience is quite common. Most students, adequately taught, attend a few classes and soon find themselves drawn back for more. A part of *tapas* is out of our control. By practicing asana we are awakening our life force, and an aspect of that energy is *tapas*. But the other part of *tapas* is entirely up to us. Vicki realizes that if she does not act on the impulse toward health that is now alive in her life, nothing more will come of it. She will have been given a glimpse of another life, and that is all. *Tapas* is also the will to realize the opportunity that is yoga, to make it real for us, to make it stick.

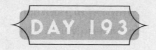

You yourselves are the Being you are seeking.

Swami Vivekananda

Something beautiful happens on the mat for the student who stays with yoga practice even for a short time. An awareness begins to dawn. Having been immersed in an outwardly focused culture, most of us come to yoga in search of something we do not have, something we cannot even name. As the weeks turn into months, though, we begin to understand that we are no longer seeking something outside ourselves, or something that we do not have. A powerful understanding starts to take shape. Our attention shifts from what we can get to who we can be. Without anyone needing to tell us—but simply by spending time on the mat with ourselves—we arrive at the conclusion that we are the ones we have been waiting for. This is the beginning of *svadhyaya,* or self-study, on the mat.

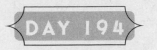

Everything that I do—when I go to workshop, when I take a class, when I teach a class—it is all part of the same learning; it is just magic. That's a lot of what yoga has brought back into my life. When I was a kid, there was a sense of magic all over the place. I used to love fairy tales. But you get into adulthood, and it's gone. There was a real hole in my heart, and that started to feel like a hole in my life. Yoga filled the hole, and it renewed my faith. There is magic, there is guidance, there is spirituality, there is God.

Natalie G., yoga teacher

I often lose sight of this. My practice becomes an obligation, a necessity, yet another thing to knock off my to-do list. When I approach my practice with this attitude, not only is it a whole lot less fun, but I am also missing the point. A fundamental principle of yoga is that the conjunction of the seer (us) with the seen (life) is intended to be educational. Our entire lives are one big lesson. In microcosm, our time spent on the mat is meant to be an exercise in self-study, or *svadhyaya*. The magic that Natalie is connecting to in her practice lies within her. The divine spark, the magic, the beauty that we yearn for are our own. This is what we are studying, and the asana are our classroom.

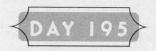

When my master and I were walking in the rain, he would say,
"Do not walk so fast, the rain is everywhere."

Shunryu Suzuki

Out of the pain of where we have been, many of us come to the mat in a hurry. Our self-study has revealed a universe of pain and loss, while at the same time it has intimated that there is a better way. Some work on the mat has brought some relief; therefore, we assume, more work on the mat will bring more relief. So we attend workshop after workshop, attempt postures of ever increasing difficulty. We are in a hurry to escape the pain we have been in and are still contending with, but our haste is self-defeating. Do not walk so fast. The pain you wish to escape is everywhere. Do not walk so fast. The grace you seek is everywhere.

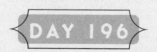

Who is the Knower that knows the world but cannot itself
be known? Who is the Hearer that hears the birds but cannot
itself be heard? Who is the Seer that sees the clouds but
cannot itself be seen?

Ken Wilber

All of the work we do on the mat comes down to this: Who are we? Why are we here? As the months become years, our asana practice reveals to us

PART THREE

Postures of Yoga

241

what we are not. We are not our fears, our desires, our thoughts, or our limitations. We begin to see that as the mind is refined, so is the body. But what does that indicate? What is the relationship between the seen and the unseen, the metaphysical mind and the physical body? This inquiry is self-study. The asana train us to identify not with what is seen but with who is seeing; not with feeling but with who is feeling. With practice, our point of reference shifts. We are no longer swayed by the light show of sensation that is the world we live in. Our focus turns inward. What began as search becomes a discovery. We come to understand that what we have been looking for is already here.

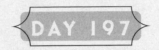

DAY 197

I had crossed the line and I was free; but there was no one to welcome me to the land of freedom. I was a stranger in a strange land.

Harriet Tubman

The final *niyama* is *isvara-pranidhana,* or surrender to God. Surrender flows naturally from the work that we do on the other *yamas* and *niyamas.* Most of us first encounter it on the mat in the form of a higher sense of purpose. We may have no idea what the *yamas* and *niyamas* are, but we find that our time spent on the mat has changed our perspective. Many of the concerns we shared with our coworkers, families, and friends simply vanish as our yoga practice gives rise to a new set of priorities. We find that we have crossed a line and are now living in a new land, but there is no one there to welcome us. Our friends or partners may laugh, and think this new obsession is just a phase. We are strangers in a strange land. But the sense of dislocation is temporary. Our roots are in new soil, and over time, a new life will grow up around us. Eventually Harriet Tubman guided three hundred other slaves to freedom and spent the remaining sixty years of her life helping freed slaves. In so doing she demonstrated how we might proceed in this new land we find ourselves in, and what surrender to God might look like.

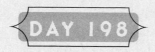

DAY 198

God is our highest instinct to know ourselves.

Deepak Chopra

Surrendering to God is surrendering to the possibility that was presented to the world when we were born. It has been established that we use very little of the potential of our brains. In asana practice we learn that we have been using very little of the potential in our bodies as well. As a species, we have a tremendous resistance to fully inhabiting the bodies and the minds God gave us. *Isvara-pranidhana* is the decision to give up this resistance.

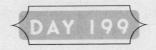

When we see our self as the center and separate from
everyone and everything else, we have to continuously
protect and guard this self.

Zen master Dennis Genpo Merzel

New students tire more readily than experienced ones. One of the easiest ways for me to convince a new, athletic student that there's something to yoga is to place her in class behind someone twenty years older than she is. Forty minutes later, the new athlete will be seated on the floor, exhausted, watching a woman old enough to be her mother breezing through her practice. The difference between the two students is obvious; one has practiced longer than the other. But what does that mean? What has the older, more experienced student learned?

With each visit to the mat we develop an ever greater efficiency and economy of movement. The muscles that need work, work; the muscles that don't need work, don't. Hence, the flowing, graceful, effortless movements of an experienced yogi. The experienced student practices with an ever increasing level of surrender. None of her energies are spent upholding or defending her sense of self. She simply does not fight against her physicality. She trusts, she breathes, she smiles into the postures as they come up, one at a time. She has learned to let go into the flow of life. Because she has come to understand her oneness with all things, her practice has become surrender in action.

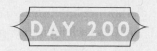

There were no promises left unbroken, no painful words unsaid.

Bonnie Raitt

I suspect I'll live the rest of my days without ever reading a more accurate summation of the beginning of my journey. As the years pass, the rawness of that moment fades. All that's left is its shadow—my reluctance to speak of my past to new friends, the skipping over of certain details, the awkward silences when I first introduced my wife-to-be to my parents.

In class, I say over and over again that our greatest liability becomes our greatest strength. Where did I learn this? A student asked a friend of mine, "How did Rolf get that way? Was he born wise?" You cannot give what you do not have. I am in the second-chance business, the get-a-new-life business. And I am not just a teacher, I am a member of the club. A man who helped me in the beginning told me I would be reborn, but that this time I would be wide awake for it, that I would witness each excruciating, exhilarating, magnificent moment. That has been true. But I first had to surrender, and to surrender I first had to be profoundly, utterly humbled. This is a tricky business. Many people die on their way to surrender. My older sister died long before she was ready to give up the fight. Part of the problem is that surrender has such a bad rap—despite the fact that the alternative is usually well documented and a lot worse. A newly sober friend told me of a family member who commented that it must be a drag to go to sober holiday parties. "No," he answered, "sober Christmas parties are not a drag. Waking up in a strange room, covered with vomit, next to someone you don't know, that's a drag."

"Surrender" is just another word for letting go. For stepping away, for stopping, for saying *enough,* for saying you are sick and tired of being sick and tired, for saying that you do not know. I have said that I did not know what was best for me, and in so doing I found out. My life did not start until I was willing to acknowledge my humanity. I took a risk. I allowed my fear of death to overcome my fear of you, and I asked for help. You have been there for me ever since. That is why it is not a drag for me to teach fifteen or twenty yoga classes a week. Teaching is a good way for me to say thank you. I will never be able to repay my debt to the ordinary people who saved my life. And that is just fine with me, because the day my debt is repaid, I will probably be done with this life. Until that day, I will continue to say thank you.

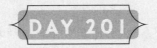

Whatever you do, even if you help somebody cross the road,
you do it to Jesus. Even giving somebody a glass of water, you
do it to Jesus. Such a simple little teaching, but it is more and
more important.

Mother Teresa

Asana practice is a study in interconnectedness. We come to see that a minor shift in the attitude of our big toes dramatically alters our experience of a posture. We practice breathing into every cell of our bodies, our eyes resting at one point, our awareness taking in all points. As our body awareness grows, our postures become an embodiment of nonviolence, an expression of faith, compassion, and honesty. To achieve this, we have had to face, and systematically deconstruct, the myriad ways in which we have chosen to be separate from our bodies. Where we have withheld love, we have had to learn to extend love. But if this lesson does not carry over into the rest of our relationships, nothing of any lasting value will have been gained. We will have failed to understand the central teaching of the asana, which is to extend love impartially. "Such a simple little teaching, but it is more and more important."

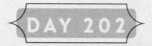

Compassion refers to the arising in the heart of the desire to relieve the suffering of all beings. At its most evolved form, compassionate action does not arise solely out of personal desire. Rather, it arises from a desire created by the collective suffering of all beings.

Ram Das

A number of students at my studio come to yoga as adolescents in adult bodies. They have been winners in the game of life, often having been blessed with the looks, opportunities, and talents associated with success in our society. The only suffering they are aware of is the bad back or bum knee they hope to straighten out with a few yoga classes. As the months turn into years, though, something changes in their faces. They begin to look me in the eye; they are in less of a hurry. As their bodies seem to grow younger, their spirits mature. I discover that this student is in the habit of giving rides to strangers from the studio; that one is providing much-needed job advice to unemployed fellow yogis; this one is volunteering. Students tell me about books they are reading that are changing their lives; they talk about their desires for their careers to be more meaningful. Eventually these yearnings are realized; their hopes come to pass. They either leave their jobs or change within them. Some leave stuck relationships; oth-

PART THREE

Postures of Yoga

247

ers finally commit and get married. Before long I am honored to know these individuals; they model virtues that I would like to embody in my own life. The externals differ, but the internal shift is the same. These men and women are surrendering to their humanity, and in so doing they are lessening the collective suffering of all beings.

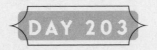

DAY 203

To put the world right in order we must first put the nation in order; to put the nation in order, we must first put the family in order; to put the family in order, we must first cultivate our personal life; we must first set our hearts right.

Confucius

Over time I've come to see my asana practice as a sort of archaeological dig. As the years pass, I unearth layer after layer of the habitual thinking that has caused me suffering. Most of it would not be considered pathological in a clinical sense. It is simply the typical thinking of my culture, class, gender, time, and space, and I have internalized all of it. As I slowly rehabilitate my physical self, peeling back layers of stiffness, musculoskeletal imbalance, scar tissue, and trauma, I am also encountering the stored memories of many lifetimes. The experience is akin to cleaning out your grandmother's attic and discovering, amongst the trunks and boxes, some clues to your family's behavior. There are many aspects to this unpacking process, but part of it, for me, is about confronting my own spiritual ignorance. My years on the mat have revealed to me, first, that I have suffered profoundly by allowing the flawed thinking of the world to define me, and second, that there has always been a part of me that has known better. I think of that part of me as sanity. Yoga practice uncovers the part of ourselves that knows better, and thereby sets our hearts right.

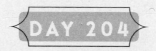

> Devotee: What are the obstacles to realization of the Self?
> Ramana Maharshi: They are the habits of the mind.
>
> *Talks with Ramana Maharshi*

Our yoga mat is a mirror. The habits of the mind that create suffering everywhere else in our lives turn up on our mats as well. It takes most of us quite a while to see that our suffering is caused by our habitual thoughts about the world, rather than by the nature of the world. There is a long process of letting go of our cherished belief that if we could only make the world a little more to our liking, everything would be just fine. Eventually we arrive at the conclusion that if we want our outsides to change, we are going to have to change our insides. Our "insides" are our thinking. More to the point, they are our habitual thinking, the stuff we think over and over again—our chronic fears, prejudices, and desires. Yoga did not invent these self-defeating habits of mind, but our ancient teachers compiled a handy list of them, which I introduced to you earlier as the five *kleshas,* or afflictions. The *kleshas*—ignorance, pride, desire, aversion, and fear of death— give us an understanding of the problems. The asana give us a chance to see the problems in action and to apply the principles of yoga to overcome them. To begin, develop the habit of noting your own habitual reactions on the mat, all of them.

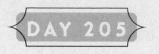

Buddha saw that suffering and evil are rooted
in a mistake about how life works.

Deepak Chopra

The first affliction, the one from which all the others flow, is our mistaken view about how life works. We do not know who we are, and therefore we make poor choices about how to proceed. According to yoga, the mistake we make is to identify with the external.

In macrocosm, this can be seen when countries struggle with past wrongdoing. Elements within French society today, for example, are unable to come to terms with the Vichy government's culpability in the death of over three hundred thousand French Jews during World War II. Identified with a false image of France, they cannot simply say, "We were dreadfully wrong, and we are terribly sorry." To do so would be to overturn their image of France, and thereby unalterably change their understanding of themselves. And so, for the last half century, there has been a concerted effort within France to deny and repress the truth of French treatment of Jewish citizens during the war.

On the personal level, we arrive on our mats identified with the results of our actions. We are good if we "win," bad if we "lose." We compete with the students to the left and right of us. We bask in the glory of a good day, are crushed by the ignominy of a bad one.

The emptiness of all this striving to control reality stems from the emptiness of our vision of who we are. The fall of Adam and Eve occurred when they began to believe that they were separate from God. Pollution, war, greed, and hate began when we stopped believing that we are one with all things. You are not your fingers or your hamstrings or this book. You are that which is understanding this book and which pervades all things. That is God, you are God, and you share God with all beings. Our time on the mat is a long journey from the idea of separation to the idea of connectedness. Our experiences on the mat, our reactions, our fears and desires are opportunities to find out who we are and who we are not.

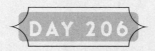

DAY 206

When the heart is right, "for" and "against" are forgotten.

Thomas Merton

The state of spiritual ignorance is fear. In the dark as to our true nature, we are afraid. So we spend our days trying to protect a self we envision as being weak and vulnerable to attack. The world is split into things that can make us feel less afraid and things that make us even more afraid. On the mat, we experience this vague fear as an inability to know peace for more than fleeting moments. At the beginning of *shavasana,* or corpse pose, we lie back and it is fine. The instructions of the teacher guide us toward a resting place. The energy of our practice swirls around us, and our body feels loose and tired in a wholesome way. Life is good. Then our fear reasserts itself: "I really should call my mother." "That was a great practice, I am finally getting it." "This was a bad practice and I am going downhill and I will be fat forever." If we're lucky, we will calm down and resettle into the peace of *shavasana.* As often as not, however, our fears are off to the races and we will simply lie there, going over the same old ground, recycling the same old fears.

This is *asmita,* an exaggerated sense of I-ness, or self-centered fear. The asana restore balance to our bodies and our spirits, and over time they address *asmita* as well. Many postures require us to be unafraid. Others require us to let go, to surrender parts of ourselves while other aspects of ourselves are being strong and expansive. Still others fold us back into ourselves. We experience ourselves over and over again—as a tree, a fish, a crow, a dog, a child, a crane. Not separate, but one with all creation. The asana slowly wear away our sense of an isolated self, as water wears away a rock. The heart settles, and "for" and "against" fade like shadows before the sun.

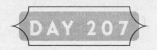

DAY 207

Now, when I'm in a situation that's a little scary or unpleasant, I can just acknowledge it. I don't have to attach to it all of the baggage that I would have attached to it before, like, "What if this happens? What if that happens?" I believe it has something to do with the way in which yoga allows me to release layers of tension or tightness. I have an image of a body that has shoulders hunched in and head down, versus a body in which the chest is open, where I can see more of what is around me. My heart feels more open now. I feel more connected to the ground I am walking on.

Gil C., yoga student

Gil is describing the experience of asana wearing away *asmita*. Over the years of his practice, Gil has arrived at a decreased sense of the isolated self and come more fully into himself. His heart is open. He is connected to the ground he walks on. I saw a movie once in which the central character slowly uncovers a medieval masterpiece that had been painted over, in the chapel of a modern-day English church. As the movie progresses, we watch the masterpiece gradually appear under the patient care of the main character. Asana practice is like that, only in yoga we are both the masterpiece and the methodical artist painstakingly working to uncover the hidden work of art.

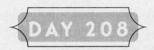

Doing your best is taking the action because you love it, not because you're expecting a reward. Most people do exactly the opposite: They only take action when they expect a reward, and don't enjoy the action. That is why they don't do their best.

Don Miguel Ruiz

The third affliction is desire. Afraid in a fearful world, we very much want certain things to happen, and we very much want certain other things not to happen. Our experience of life is like that of a trapeze artist—but instead of rings, we swing from one intense attachment to the next. We begin asana practice with an eye to the results. We've heard that stretching is good for the back, or helps with stress, and so we "go to yoga" to get a little something we feel we are lacking. This consumer attitude serves the purpose of getting us to the mat in the first place, but it must be abandoned if we are to stay there. This is especially so because the first year of asana practice often produces spectacular results. Years of pain vanish, diseases reverse themselves, body image problems fade, a whole new world is presented to us. Why not hope for more of the same? Because it is in this hoping that we lose sight of the true beauty we have discovered.

Asana practice is an immersion into the now. The work we do on the mat teaches us to commit wholeheartedly to the present moment. We act in the moment with all our hearts because we are learning that that is all there is. We are finding that the only result worth achieving is being here now. All other positive outcomes are by-products of our present-moment awareness. To be attached to the results, be they a tighter bum or a better triangle pose, is to place the cart before the horse and to miss the point. Eventually we will find this striving unrewarding. And then we will put our mats on the shelf to collect dust, alongside all the other devices we've used in the hope of achieving specific results. The alternative—doing your best as an expression of your love for life—is the path that leads to a long and fulfilling asana practice.

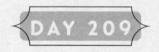

DAY 209

What we need to do is to recognize Inner Nature and work with Things As They Are. When we don't, we get into trouble.

Benjamin Hoff

Desire is the wish for things to be not as they are. What is wrong with that? In a culture that reveres progress, working with things as they are sounds depressingly like fatalism. Did Martin Luther King Jr. work with things as they are? Did Helen Keller work with things as they are? Did Rocky? Well, yes, they did, actually. Dwelling in the real, individuals who accomplish great deeds demonstrate what is possible, demonstrate how things are. There is nothing fatalistic about working with things as they are. Fatalism begins when we leave the present, when we forsake the real in favor of our imaginations. Within the real lie the seeds of all our dreams. As we accept and connect with the postures that are hard for us, we find the understanding that leads to mastery. That is working with things as they are.

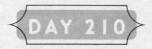

> The disciples of any religious system can say we are good
> and the others, those that are not like us, the sinners,
> they are bad. This can be exhilarating to the souls of
> toxically shamed persons.
>
> John Bradshaw

There is a back to every front. Desire and aversion are two sides of the same coin. Both have the ability to move us deeply, to take us completely out of ourselves, to lead us into behavior that we later cannot recognize as our own. As an active addict, my desire for the relief provided by alcohol or other drugs caused me to spend ten years of my life as a person I can hardly recognize. Photographs from that time depict a person fundamentally different from who I was before my addiction and from who I am now. Aversion is no less powerfully intoxicating. The staggering atrocities of the twentieth century and the horrifying terrorism of the twenty-first are all attributable to aversion. In the microcosm of the yoga mat, aversion plays a more subtle role, but it remains an intoxicant—as the teacher who is a distraction, or the postures we do not attempt, or the barely concealed contempt we express when describing a different style of yoga.

We spend our lives riding a wave of resentment and aversion that is so close to the surface that even the innocent person placing his mat too close to ours is enough to trigger it. Because we do not want to admit how angry

PART THREE

Postures of Yoga

we are, how out of control we are, we cannot do anything about it. Without a radically new definition of who we are, this unfortunate state is permanent. The breath and the postures allow us to systematically redefine who we are. The breath calms the mind and draws it inward, severing its ties to desire and aversion. The postures deconstruct our old definitions of self. We walk on new feet, see with new eyes, experience life from the inside out. Note aversion as it arises, but do not try to control the uncontrollable. Let go of the problem and embrace the solution with all your heart.

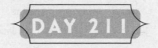

DAY 211

An attack thought or a hostile thought will create a buildup of
energy in the body that we call anger. . . . The more you are
identified with your thinking, your likes and dislikes, judgments
and interpretations, which is to say the less present you are as
the watching consciousness, the stronger the emotional energy
charge will be, whether you are aware of it or not.

Eckhart Tolle

The first form of courage I learned was physical courage. By the time I was jumping out of airplanes for the army, I had learned to detach from my thoughts about my own physical safety. In fact, I'd cultivated clear seeing to the point that only my first jump was memorable. Subsequent jumps were no big deal; they warranted very little emotional energy. My yoga practice has brought me in touch with an entirely different sort of courage. Being disliked for doing the right thing, not getting my way, being viewed by others as inadequate—these and a host of other circumstances all seem like less of a big deal than they used to. Where my fragile ego used to collapse under judgment and criticism, I now find myself expending less and less emotional energy worrying about what others think of me.

The asana bring with them a myriad of circumstances that trigger emotional responses. Is there a yoga student alive who can't identify with this one, for example: "I am afraid this moronic teacher will have us in this posture forever, and I will look weak by coming out of it before the rest of the class. I fervently desire to get the heck out of this posture." As our practice matures, though, we begin to realize that strong emotional responses merely cloud the mind and exhaust the body. Through clear seeing, we come to understand the roots of these responses and learn to let them go. Pride, fear, and desire slowly fade.

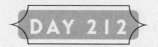

Love of fame, love of power, stimulate men to most strenuous effort. But when they are grasped and held in the hand, weariness is the result. . . . Does God mock us with all the objects [of our desire]? No. The object has been to bring about the power of the Self, to develop the capacity latent in man.

Annie Besant

In the beginning we desire the fruits of a good practice. Early on, we are afraid of falling over in balancing postures and looking foolish in class. Desire and aversion stimulate us to work hard. Eventually we experience neither desire nor aversion, we just practice.

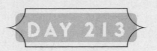

In the absence of knowing the infinite source of energy and creativity, life's miseries come into being. Getting close to God through true knowledge heals the fear of death, confirms the existence of the soul, and gives ultimate meaning to life.

Deepak Chopra

Deepak Chopra captures the essence of the *kleshas,* including the final *klesha, abhinivesa,* or fear of death. The fact that we can work to allay our fear of death by practicing yoga postures might at first seem far-fetched. And what exactly is our fear of death anyway? This morning my dog disturbed a particularly vengeful hive of hornets. My dog, my wife, and I ran like the dickens. Is that fear of death? I believe our fear is so all-pervasive that we have difficulty even seeing it. On the mat, it manifests as our grasping desire for more, better, faster yoga postures. It manifests in our restlessness, our difficulty in *shavasana.* It is the prevailing sense that we are not doing enough, and that we won't get there, wherever "there" is. My own fear of death is so general that only in its absence do I even become aware of it. I catch a glimpse of such peace when I can allow my body and my postures to be imperfect, when I can simply let things be as they are. In class I remind students that swimmers who fight against the water tire and drown. Those who relax into it float. It is like that with us and God. On our mats we learn to float.

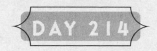

> In the absence of knowing the infinite source of energy and creativity, life's miseries come into being. Getting close to God through true knowledge heals the fear of death, confirms the existence of the soul, and gives ultimate meaning to life.
>
> Deepak Chopra

I repeat this quote because it tells us so much about the reason we fear death and what we are meant to do about it in our yoga practice. We are afraid because we have drawn away from God. We will be unafraid when we draw near. How do we do this on the mat? Well, begin by doing what you are already doing. You are firm and relaxed, which implies that you are noting tension. You are becoming familiar with what body workers call "cringing patterns," your habitual protective tension. Day after day, you are becoming adept at releasing ever deeper and more subtle layers of tension, while still maintaining the posture. You are learning to trust. Trust is the opposite of *abhinivesa*. Let your asana practice be an exploration in trust.

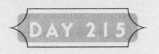

The mind is restless, unsteady, turbulent, wild and stubborn:
truly, it seems to me as hard to master as the wind.

Bhagavad Gita

Walking down a forest path, or practicing asana on a late afternoon, our minds can be still. We are one with the breath, one with the moment, one with all things; there is peace and joy, oneness. Then our minds click back into gear and we are transported into another realm. The injustices at work must be sorted out, our fears and desires must be explored once again, and suddenly we feel the familiar pain of separation; the beauty of the walk or our practice is not even a memory.

Our training can bring us back into the moment. Once again we are on the path in the woods, a shining vision; once again we are on the mat, a possibility is realized. These are the two realms we travel between. The *kleshas* merely catalogue the afflictions of a false world. Our practice trains us to live in the real one.

The mind is as hard to master as the wind. If we try to outthink it, or to figure it out, we will forever be like a dog chasing its tail. We are on the forest path, or in the late-afternoon practice; the mind wanders, and we gently bring it back. That is all. The other world, the world of the *kleshas,* the world in which we wage a perpetual war against reality, is not real. We note it and return to the real. There is nothing to master because there is nothing there.

DAY 216

Have you ever noticed how eager young children are to learn about everything? And how they are constantly moving while doing so? Whether they are painting at an easel, stirring cake batter, or building blocks, their whole body is involved. And learning occurs during this movement.

Maureen Murdock

A yoga posture is a whole-body experience. As my practice deepens, this awareness deepens as well. Are the muscles of my face and neck relaxed? What is the attitude of my lips? What am I doing with my toes? Is there violence present in the way I maintain the posture? Fear? Desire? Greed? Does the breath flow freely to all parts of my body, or is it blocked by unnecessary tension? Do I deepen the posture through contraction, or release? The inquiry is ever expanding. The inquiry is childlike; it is the movement of consciousness; it is wisdom in action.

> # ⟨ DAY 217 ⟩

> Goals and contingencies, as I've said, are important. But they
> exist in the future and the past, beyond the pale of the sensory
> realm. Practice, the path of mastery, exists only in the present.
>
> George Leonard

Like most people, I am actually galvanized by a goal. As I write these words, I am also getting ready for the photo shoot for this book and preparing to open a new yogo studio. Both events are occasions for me to deepen my practice. There is an excitement as I prepare for the big game. (Of course, there is no big game, but old habits die hard.) I work harder, and more often, when I feel that I am getting ready for something. I plan my practice schedule and organize my week around it. Then it's show time. All of my plans and goals, my hopes and dreams, come down to the next two or three hours. Can I overcome my resistance to hard work? Can I get to the place where it all comes together, where I am glad to be doing exactly what I need to be doing? Each practice is its own mountain to climb. Each practice brings us back to the importance of *now*. Our achievements are simply the by-products of our ability to realize the potential of the present moment. That is what we are here to learn. That is the juice.

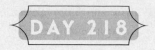

DAY 218

If your eyes and ears are open, you will see the windows of opportunity open around you.

Cherie Carter-Scott

In asana our eyes are open, our ears are open, our minds are open, our hearts are open. As the months turn into years, we realize that our practice is a long unfolding, an opening into promise. We learn to stand easy, firm, and relaxed, and our problems become the open windows of opportunity.

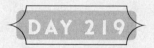

DAY 219

True men of Yoga, striving, see Him within themselves.

Bhagavad Gita

Success in asana requires stamina. I forget this in times when I am not working very hard at my practice, and I remember it when I am. If I train hard and long enough, usually over the course of a few months, something magical happens. I find that in posture after posture, I can endure past the initial difficulty. The pain softens, and the training of my mind begins to kick in. I invite myself to relax, to breathe, to enter the dance of the asana, mind, body, and breath. I encourage myself to have faith, to smile, to have fun, to feel gratitude, to be in love with the moment, the opportunity, the posture. This requires strength, physical endurance, and mental discipline. The fruit of this strength, this discipline, is that I am able to pause in each posture and connect to life pulsing in every cell of my body—life dancing in me, life dancing through me.

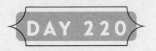

DAY 220

In the night of all beings, the wise man sees only
the radiance of the Self.

Bhagavad Gita

I have found that the asana are an answer to the difficulty of our times. Certainly I have not been above the darkness of our times, the "night of all beings." On the contrary, I have known its depths. I have spent more days in this lifetime with despair in my heart than hope. But yoga brings me in touch with the light. One of the qualities of this light is the knowledge that if we have our soul, we have everything, and if we lose it, we have nothing. Yoga connects us to our soul. Our practice reminds us that we already have everything that we need. Amidst the unspeakable sorrows and injustices of the material world, we find the endless brilliance of the spirit. Our connection to our own soul serves as a reminder to those around us, clearing the way for them to reconnect to spirit themselves. In the night of all beings, our practice is a radiant light.

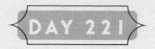

You can't think about presence, and the mind can't understand
it. Understanding presence is being present.

Eckhart Tolle

Lately my asana practice is giving me the distinct experience of moving
through layers of stored memory. In the same half hour I might be deeply
connected to memories of my early twenties, then pulled further back, to
the emotional reality of my middle school years, then rushed forward again
to my mid-twenties. I have the sense that, after many years of practice, I am
reclaiming a command over my physicality that was lost through chemical
addiction. For me, it is like coming full circle. There is a sense of reclama-
tion mixed together with layers of emotion that seem to span all of this lifetime and maybe more. I have learned to trust this process, despite the fact
that I do not fully understand it or know where it is leading me, because
within it I feel God and a sense of my own fulfillment. My practice is not a
place I understand; rather, it is a place that I go.

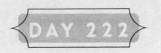

Mature in yoga, impartial everywhere that he looks, he sees
himself in all beings and all beings in himself.

Bhagavad Gita

On Labor Day weekend, my wife and I spent an evening on Main Street in Northampton, Massachusetts, eating frozen yogurt and watching the people walk by. I have been visiting this town since I was in my early twenties and have shared almost all of the most significant events of my life with this place. A number of my ancestors lie buried across the valley, in Amherst.

Over the years, my spiritual condition has been reflected in how I've viewed the people out for an evening stroll. On this evening, I love them all. I was not prepared for this. Like most of us, I've been afflicted by judgment. Tonight, though, judgment has lost its grip on me. We pass a lesbian couple whose joy touches me unexpectedly, as if they are my sisters and I've been forever enriched by their happiness. Teenagers, then parents and their young children, go by. We pass couples, singles, gangs, and groups, and I love them all. Yoga encourages us to connect to what is real, and what is real is love.

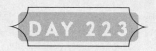

DAY 223

The man who sees me in everything, and everything within me,
will not be lost to me, nor will I ever be lost to him.

Bhagavad Gita

In class I say we practice yoga at the intersection of energy, matter, and consciousness. Asana is the place where physical and metaphysical meet. We breathe at the edge of two worlds, and over time, we come to see that they are one. My practice has given me the ability to experience life with a quiet mind. When my mind is quiet, I can see spirit in everything, and I know that everything, naturally, is contained in spirit. When my mind is distracted, though, I am lost to this precious awareness. So I practice, alive to the diversity of energy, matter, and consciousness, and in order to perceive the unity of the all-encompassing spirit. What a beautiful thing, to walk amidst the endless diversity of life with the ability to perceive the source and the reality of its unity.

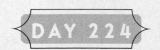

DAY 224

He who is rooted in oneness realizes that I am in every being:
Wherever he goes, he remains in me.

Bhagavad Gita

I read once that a great sage said the whole world was his home. It has stayed with me, this idea that we can so transcend our fear and our sense of separateness that we would feel at home wherever we went. This is an extremely nourishing vision for me. It is also the direction we are moving in as we learn to be at home in the asana. We enter a posture, and we let go of the need to resist, the assumption that we do not belong. We relax, we breathe, we explore, we make ourselves at home. Off the mat, we encounter another being—a spider, a person we love, a person we do not know—and we let go of the need to react, to feel separate. We relax, breathe, explore what it is to be in relationship. We allow ourselves to be at home. This process must begin in our hearts, for we suffer from loneliness because we believe we are alone. To end this suffering, we embrace a new belief. We become rooted in oneness, in the idea that we are all love, and love is all there is.

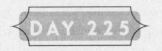

When he sees all beings as equals in suffering or in joy because they are like himself, that man has grown perfect in yoga.

Bhagavad Gita

Like a Polaroid photo coming slowly into focus, the aim of our practice reveals itself to us. By the time I was five or six, I think I had already been driven mad by the collective fear of the world. I lied, I cheated, and I stole to protect a self I saw as isolated and unsafe. By the time I began a genuine spiritual practice, I had grown tired of my fear but I knew nothing else. The first messages that got through to me were that I no longer had to hurt myself and that I no longer needed to be afraid. This came as an indescribable relief. The photograph in this book of me in child pose speaks to this. In meditation and on the mat I have slowly deconstructed my physical, mental, and spiritual fear. What occurs in the absence of fear? Love.

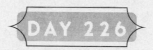

Note: When Neena began practicing yoga, she was suffering from a chronic thyroid condition and a shoulder injury that her doctors told her would never completely heal.

> Within two months after my first yoga class, my arm was completely healed. About that time, I told my doctor that I was going to stop taking the thyroid pills I had been sentenced to for the rest of my life. We agreed to monitor my blood every three months. After the first three months, I was within spec— barely. My doctor thought I should go back on the pills, but I asked her for another three months. At my next checkup, my blood tests indicated that my thyroid was completely normal. It has stayed that way since. Reversal of this condition is quite rare. My doctor was amazed but she didn't attribute it to yoga. I know, however, that I didn't change anything else in my life. It *had* to be yoga.
>
> Neena, yoga student

Neena's story is particularly dramatic, but all of us have similar stories of our own and are familiar with many more. What, exactly, happens when we practice asana? Why these remarkable recoveries for which Western medicine has no explanation? The simplest answer has to do with *prana,* or life force. The asana unblock blocked life force. Neena's story can be understood as a remarkable instance of a person's life force reasserting itself. The reassertion of life force will be different for each one of us, but the overall effect is the same—abundant mental, physical, and spiritual health. This explanation works for me, but as a teacher and a student I have often wondered at the mechanics of these miracles. The key seems to be in the fact that the asana force us to act as a coordinated whole—mind, body, and spirit. Individually and collectively we suffer from alienation. Our minds are split off from parts of our bodies, our souls are disconnected from our hearts, the privileged in our society are split off from the nonprivileged. Yoga in general, and asana specifically, is a program of forced integration. Today, simply observe the experience of residing in a posture as an integrated whole—mind, body, and spirit.

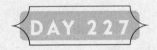

You may not be what you think you are,
but what you think, you are.

Jim Clark

To understand the asana at work on our bodies we must first arrive at an understanding of our physicality. Despite the fact that most of us have not taken formal anatomy and physiology courses, we are still the inheritors of Western medicine's understanding of the human body. Like all institutions, Western medicine reflects the political and economic systems within which it has existed. The emphasis has been placed on things being separate—this is mine, that is yours. This muscle begins here and ends there. This bone begins here and ends there. This organ performs this discrete function with this discrete result, and if there is a problem with the attainment of the result, we "fix" this discrete organ. Nautilus weight training equipment is a product of this kind of thinking. As these machines showed up in health clubs and gyms across the country, much was made of the fact that this equipment could isolate a specific muscle group and exercise it throughout its range of motion. No thought was given to the fact that training like this would, over time, develop some muscles and not others, leading to unnatural imbalance and injury.

Western medicine is based on the assumption that the body is made up of separate parts, like a machine. But we can begin to understand the power of the asana only when we come to see the body as an integrated, balance-seeking whole. Our practice is an in-depth exploration into the reality of this conception of the body. Notice the moments in your practice when you experience yourself as an integrated whole. Notice the moments when your tendency is to do otherwise. Note when one side of the body over-powers the other, when you do violence to one aspect of your body in an attempt to open or lengthen another. Begin to see your practice as a search for balanced and integrated effort.

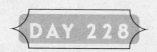

DAY 228

Know ye not that your bodies are the members of Christ?

I Corinthians 6:15

For years I practiced yoga without really understanding how it was that my body incorporated the truths revealed in asana practice. When a skilled body worker began attending my classes, we started to work together. His understanding of the body revealed to me a holistic model that was in keeping with my own intuitive work on the mat.

The body, as my friend explained, is shaped and contained by an all-encompassing web of connective tissue. As the world is held together by divine consciousness, so the body is held together by connective tissue. Lao-Tzu provided us a clue into our internal universe when he wrote, "Empty yet inexhaustible, it gives birth to infinite worlds." Connective tissue is not only the fabric that holds us together; it's the substance that gives shape to the innumerable spaces within the body, the many worlds of our organs, bones, nerves, and vascular system.

The work I did with my friend explored the long, integrated lines of connective tissue running the length of my body. We each experience these lines in the sweep and swirl of the asana. As I grew to understand the role of this web of connective tissue in my body, I saw in it the key to understanding the mechanics of the miracles we experience on the mat. I also began to glimpse a profound relationship between our spiritual reality and our physical reality.

Connective tissue then, in its various shapes and consistencies, forms a continuous net throughout the entire body. It contains many specialized structures, but it is really all one piece, from scalp to soles and from skin to marrow. If all the other tissues were extracted, the connective framework alone would preserve the three dimensional human form in all its details.

Deane Juhan

Connective tissue, like consciousness, expands and contracts. In asana we work to expand the connective tissue. Rather like a plastic bag that has been stretched, the connective tissue contracts again, but not to its original dimensions. The progressive nature of this lengthening and expanding process over time explains why such amazing feats of flexibility are possible, and why no amount of stiffness is reason for despair. For today, just begin to experience your practice at the level of your connective tissue. Arriving on your mat, you first encounter your connective tissue as limiting and stiff. Then, as you move deeper into the practice, it warms and softens; expansive openings are available to you that you could not achieve even a half hour before. At the end of practice, your body feels loose and comfortable. Your entire system of connective tissue, the organ that defines your physical form, has been expanded and filled with oxygen and life. In this process you are both the sculpture and the sculptor.

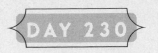
A
S
A
N
A

Janusirsasana has two major lines of energy. . . . The first major
line travels up the spine and out the crown of your head. The
second major line travels down the extended leg and outward
through the foot.

Erich Schiffmann

Erich Schiffmann is describing the point at which the most recent discoveries in body work intersect with the ancient wisdom of asana. Body workers
are now assessing the bodies of their clients in terms of lines of connective
tissue. Head-to-knee pose, or *janusirsasana,* a seated-forward bend, engages
what is called the superficial back line. This line runs from the bottom of
the feet all the way up the back, over the top of the head, and ends at the
brow. In body work terms, this posture opens the superficial back line quite
nicely. In addition to the superficial back line, we work in our postures to
open the superficial front line, the lateral line, the spiral line, and the deep
front line. An understanding of these lines reveals the brilliance of the asana
and suggests the sequence in which postures might be best performed to
open the body.

A simple way to experience this concept today would be to include sun
salutations in your warm-ups. A sun salutation alternates between opening
our superficial front line (upward dog) and opening our superficial back line
(downward dog). The back line, which is opened in forward bends, begins
at the bottom of the feet. The front line, which is opened in back bends,
begins at the tops of the feet. Connect to the sweep of these long lines in
your body today, and to their origins in your feet.

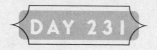

DAY 231

Two people have been living in you all your life.

Sogyal Rinpoche

Let's begin with the superficial front line, opened in back bends, and the superficial back line, which is opened in forward bends. The back line extends from the bottom of the feet all the way up the back, over the top of the head, and down to the brow. Downward dog opens the superficial back line in its entirety. In the Iyengar tradition, the brow is placed on the floor in the deepest expression of downward dog. The superficial front line extends from the tops of your feet to the sternocleidomastoids, or large muscles at the front of your neck. In upward dog the tops of your feet are on the floor; as your body opens, you will be able to safely lift the crown of your head up and back. This brings the extension of upward dog into the large muscles in the front of the neck, opening the front line in its entirety. These postures are exquisite evidence of the interplay of these lines of connective tissue, and of right alignment in a posture.

The front line and the back line also serve to bring our attention to all that is in front of us and all that is behind us. As we learn to manipulate these two aspects of ourselves, we begin to see the deeper possibilities within our practice. The back must be strong in order for the front to open; the front must hold steady for the back to open. Front and back, light and shadow, the one thing comes to us as two.

PART THREE

Postures of Yoga

275

DAY 232

The clinical and treatment implications of the deep front line
are so profound and diverse as to have already spawned several
books. . . . (The deep front line) represents the interface
between the 'gut body' and the neuromotor chassis. . . .
The connections of healthy communication along this line
to breathing, circulation, digestion, elimination, and sexual
maturity are so vast, and manifest so individually, that we are
reduced to pointing out the area, and urging practitioners
to study and feel their way into a sensitive manner of freeing,
easing, and lengthening the myriad aspects of the deep front
line. In self-development terms, the yogic back bend is the most
effective way to reach the deep front line.

Thomas Myers

The deep front line is the place in our physiology in which the aspect we
have control over, the muscular-skeletal system, connects to the aspect we
don't, our internal organs. The deep front line travels up from our base,
up the inseam of our legs, and into the world of our soft internal organs.
It moves through the structural supports that hold those organs in place,
and it makes such bodily functions as eating and verbal communication
possible. While gravity shortens and compresses the deep front line, back
bends open it. That we are actually able to free, ease, and lengthen this
line in back bends is dramatic evidence of the potency of asana. Shakespeare wrote, "We know who we are, but know not what we might
become." And so it is as we begin to open and lengthen our deep front
line. The inclusion of a sequence of back bends in your daily practice

inaugurates a profound change in your own physical destiny. With this change comes a host of positive challenges. You are rewriting history.

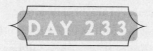

> The collagenous net (connective tissue) is to animals what cellulose is to plants—the scaffolding around which everything else is built, hung, or inserted. The major difference is that plant cellulose maximizes stability over movement, whereas collagen (connective tissue) favors mobility—with the price being a more dynamic stability. Our stability requires near-constant maintenance.
>
> Thomas Myers

Unlike plants, which put down roots and grow in place, human beings are made to move. We live out a more dynamic fate. As visionary anatomist and body worker Thomas Myers observes, "our stability requires near-constant maintenance." This appears to be true at every level of our existence. On the mat we can make use of this understanding by making stability our aim. Instead of focusing on gaining strength or flexibility in your postures, cultivate stability instead. The demands of stability will create strength, and the peace of stability will encourage exploration, equanimity, length, and surrender.

Asana isn't just a muscular effort. It is much more about taking
one's attention and spreading it throughout the whole net of
connective tissue. Every fiber, every cell becomes a part of the
mind, or realized, or remembered as a part of the mind.

David Kennedy

David Kennedy, the body worker who deepened my understanding of our physicality, introduced me to the idea of the body as a single organism, enveloped from head to toe by fascia, pliable bands of connective tissue that separate or bind together our muscles, organs, and other soft structures. Thus we begin to see the asana in a new light, as a level of consciousness that we bring to bear on the ubiquitous whole of this fibrous net.

B. K. S. Iyengar asks, "Where does the body end and the mind begin? Where does the mind end and the spirit begin? They cannot be divided, as they are interrelated and but different aspects of the same all-pervading divine consciousness."

Steady and relaxed, we breathe into the whole—mind, body, and spirit in alignment.

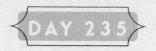

DAY 235

Where is the literature which gives expression to Nature?

Henry David Thoreau

Within each of us is the ability to spiral into a posture like a vine spiraling up a trellis. The blueprint for this magnificent movement is in the spiral line. The spiral line is a continuous line of connective tissue that begins at the arch of the foot, runs up the front of the leg, and travels once around the body, ascending as it goes, coming to rest at the base of the skull behind the ear, on the same side as the arch from which it came. There is a corresponding line that begins at the opposite arch and spirals up to the ear on that side. We experience these lines in the twisting postures. Twisting triangle is a dramatic expression of the spiral line. Anchored in the rear foot, the posture follows the spiral line and ends with the neck turning upward to bring the gaze high.

In the twisting postures we surrender to a spiral that we see duplicated throughout nature—in the lazy spiraling flight of a fly, the spin of a tornado, the undulations of vines. This spiral is also in the connective tissues that give form to our bodies. As we become at home in twisting postures, we are able to simply let them happen—they are an idea, a spiraling energy, an aspect of nature that our bodies were created to express.

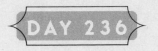

ASANA

Asana is a good example of the fact that all yogic practices are
interconnected and one step penetrates the other, the main aim
always being the concentration of the mind.

Georg Feuerstein

Yoga presents us with a bewildering array of practices and priorities. We
appear to need two days—one to prepare ourselves for life and one for living it. The truth is simpler, and the simplicity we need in order to make
headway can be found in our relationships. It is in relationships that we sow
either the seeds of our liberation or the seeds of our imprisonment. Yoga is
asking us to pay attention to the nature of all of our relationships and to
apply the *yamas* and the *niyamas* to them. Whether it is our relationship to
our breath, the bottoms of our feet, the ant crawling across the kitchen
floor, our families, or to God, we are being asked to pay attention. The aim
of yogic practice is to free us from the endless distractions of the *kleshas*—
fear, pride, desire, and ignorance—and to teach us to bring a focused mind
to bear on the nature of our relationships. Our time spent on the mat is
dedicated to that end.

DAY 237

The effect of asana is to put an end to the dualities or differentiation between the body and mind, mind and soul. None of the
pairs of opposites can exist for the *sadhaka* (practitioner) who
is one with the body, mind, and soul.

B. K. S. Iyengar

The Yoga Sutras tell us that the asana deconstruct the disconnection we feel
from ourselves, God, and one another. I believe that we each possess an
intuition toward health that can be awakened and developed by authentic
spiritual practice. This intuition is an intrinsic aspect of consciousness and it
is present in all living things. We are born with it, we can be taught to ignore
it, and we can learn to reconnect to it. Once we begin to reconnect to our
own intuition toward health, we can see it and speak to it in others. This
insight, the spiritual connectedness we recognize in others, supports and
develops our own. This is true because we are all one. And this is why group
practice is so powerful. There is an unmistakable, potent energy at work in a
yoga class, a group meditation, a roomful of people worshiping together.
The infinite diversity of life masks the underlying unity. And yet, the wave
that flows gently over my foot is not separate from the ocean. As we breathe
into a posture, steady and relaxed, with our attention embracing the totality
of our experience, we are awakening this understanding. We are all one.

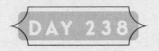
Asana practice has been a wonderful through line for me
because it's a way of embodying that work with attention, a way
of spreading attention throughout the whole of the system, and
a way of reflecting the perennial nature of life. You arrive back
at the mat day in and day out, and yet you're not the same
person you were the last time you were on the mat. Millions of
cells have come and gone, different food has been metabolized
on all different levels, whether it's food of thought, food of
emotions, food of light and energy, food of relationships, food
of organic substances. So there is all this different play in
consciousness occurring each time we practice. And then there
is the beautiful metaphor of it, training one's consciousness to
absorb multiple lifetimes within this lifetime.

David Kennedy

Consciousness is like a person on a riverbank, and life is like the river, flowing endlessly by, forever re-creating itself, forever reinventing itself. Our asana
practice provides us with a steady place from which to observe the river and
the vision to see it as it is. But there is more—we are both the sculptor and
the sculpture, the observer and the river. We come to the mat with a narrowly defined physicality. Our practice breaks down this definition and
makes possible a fluidity that is in keeping with the true nature of our existence. Each new physical reality on the mat gives birth to a corresponding
psychological and spiritual possibility, so that we flow from birth to death,
death to rebirth, endlessly re-creating ourselves, endlessly reinventing ourselves.

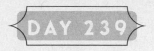

An aspirant should practice before five o'clock in the morning.

Sri K. Pattabhi Jois

I have practiced yoga from four to six in the morning, while working nine to five. The effect was great. By six-fifteen in the morning I was wide awake, having completed a thorough asana practice. I would get on a seven-fifteen bus to work feeling tremendously well prepared for the day. I was working then with the homeless mentally ill at a state mental health facility in downtown Boston, and when I walked onto the ward each morning the world was my oyster. The drawbacks were as follows: A) getting home at five-thirty and going to bed at nine on a regular basis was problematic, especially since I was also moonlighting as a yoga teacher in those days, and B) I am awfully stiff that early in the morning, and so I had trouble going very deep in my postures.

I have also practiced yoga in the late afternoon and early evening. I find that I am far more supple then, and so I'm able to work harder longer and to explore more deeply. Afterward it's late, I have a light dinner, there are no big wows. The drawbacks are as follows: A) I often spend a part of the day dreading/debating the merits of my late afternoon session, and B) a late-in-the-day practice does not serve the same purpose as an early-morning practice. An early-morning practice sets you up for the day. An afternoon practice, by default, must be an end in and of itself. The point is, there is no "perfect" time to practice, but there is an auspicious time in the day for you to practice. And when is that? You just have to figure it out for yourself.

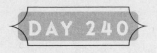

DAY 240

Sometimes more is more.

Baron Baptiste

When I have the time and energy to deepen my asana practice I sometimes do two sessions in the same day. In the morning I focus on waking up slowly and enjoying the process, preparing my body and mind for the day. Later, I may take a walk or a bike ride as a way to warm up. Then, in the afternoon or early evening, my aim in the second practice is to go long and deep. Sometimes I play music during this session. I start off slowly and build gradually. I include new postures or postures that I'm working on but don't always make time for. At the end I give myself a long time in *shavasana*. Afterwards, I treat myself to a movie with my wife, or dinner with friends, or something else that I find particularly delightful.

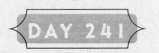

DAY 241

I think it's important not to overlook the joy of the journey due to an excess of goal orientation.

Lama Surya Das

Some of my best practices occur when, for some reason, I cannot take it to the limit. Perhaps I'm pressed for time, or I've trained a lot recently and this is a rest day, or I'm just in the mood to relax and take it easier than usual. On these days my inner coach lets up. Within me lives a coach who has prepared me for state wrestling tournaments, Army Ranger school, and more than one marathon. This individual is usually waiting for me when I arrive on my mat. He wears a whistle and a stopwatch and he consults a clipboard frequently. In his day, he was the best; even now he is usually wise and fair, but he never lets up. On those days when he knocks off early, though, I play. I do only the postures that feel really good and are fun. Every day on the mat is a small miracle, but on these days I remember how much I love my practice.

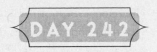

DAY 242

My soul is restless until it rests in you.

Saint Augustine

Why this emphasis placed on sustained attention? Well, what is the alternative? Spend a little quiet time today pondering the past or the future. As you do this, get a sense of your internal state. No doubt your emotions will follow the ebb and flow of your thoughts, with happy memories producing good feelings and unhappy ones giving rise to bad feelings. The emotions are authentic, but the circumstances are contrived. Floating on a sea of fantasy, our emotional lives are held captive to the endless soap operas produced by our vivid imaginations. All of the practices of yoga are aimed at ending this bondage to an imagined reality.

Now, spend a little time being really connected to something you love. Give your full attention to your family, your work, your body floating in asana. Grounded in the real, how do you feel? You may feel sad, you may feel afraid, but however you feel, you can trust that these feelings are based on reality. Sustained attention, like endurance to the marathon runner, allows us to show up for the things that matter. Anchored in the real, we can evolve and grow. The problems of our lives can be worked through, and as we do this work, in the present moment, our souls find peace.

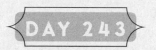

Most of the time I'm looking outside of myself to have my world view corroborated. The beauty of yoga is that when we become energetically alive, and our mind becomes drawn into direct experience of the moment, we turn inside; it's a new doorway, a new infinite world of possibilities. . . . The doorway to insight is the present moment. So the question is, how do I enter the present moment? For that, the body is an incredible tool.

Sudhir Jonathan Foust

Yogis—explorers and adventurers at heart—choose to explore the body. Instead of sailing to distant lands or encountering new species of animals or far-off peoples, yogis explore the aspect of God's creative genius that is closest at hand. One of the first things we encounter when we decide to follow in the footsteps of the yogis who have gone before us is that the body resides in the present. If we want to make any headway in our practice, we must be present enough to hear our teacher and apply her instructions. Sweating through a demanding yoga class, we are bound to the moment by our body's requirement for guidance. A posture simply won't happen on its own. We must pay attention to the alignment of our feet, our knees, our hips, our spine, our shoulders, our gaze, and our breath. Initially, all this is bewildering, and most new students tire easily. Then, as the weeks turn into months, the body becomes more supple and, at the same time, stronger. We gain new levels of physical endurance, which correspond to our increasing mental endurance. The mind is developing the ability to stay in a posture, to stay in the moment. As this ability deepens, we find that we are able to function on a different plane in everyday life. We are able to stay with a difficult situation, to hold our attention on something in spite of emotional upset. Both pleasant and unpleasant circumstances receive more of our attention. We find that in deepening our relationship to our bodies, we also deepen our relationship to reality.

DAY 244

The art of resting the mind and the power of dismissing
from it all care and worry is probably one of the secrets
of our great men.

Captain J. A. Hatfield

Throughout our practice, our mind wanders, we become distracted, we feel fatigued, and then we remember and we begin again. We come into the now. We feel and hear our breathing, we feel the air on our skin, our attention opens to encompass the experience of our entire body, we see what we are looking at, we are conscious of our heartbeat slowing, we are practicing asana. Then our mind wanders, we fatigue, we remember, and we begin again.

Over time, we come to associate a distracted mind with fatigue, anger, desire, resentment, and sorrow. We come to see the present as a refuge from the pain of our imaginations. We come to see that the present is the place where love lives. We develop the habit of a restful, focused mind. At the end of our practice we take this restful mind to a deeper level. In *shavasana,* or corpse pose, we practice profound stillness. Using the same patient willingness to begin again, we deepen our ability to rest. We do not differentiate between rest and work, we are still in action, alert in rest.

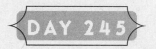

DAY 245

Blessed are the flexible for they shall not be bent out of shape.
Michael McGriffy, M.D.

By the end of my first week of yoga practice, my life had changed profoundly. Within a month, most of us are unrecognizable to ourselves. For a long time, I gave no thought to why this would be. I had stopped drinking, and that had changed my world so dramatically that moving to Mars would have been more subtle. So why shouldn't this "yoga thing" not have the same remarkable effect?

Years of teaching yoga and watching such transformations in others have given me pause to consider the profound impact a little "stretching" seems to have on the average person. Lao-Tzu wrote, "Whoever is stiff and inflexible is a disciple of death. Whoever is soft and yielding is a disciple of life." And each day I see the truth of these words dramatized in my classroom. The rigidity with which we see ourselves, our lives, everything, is manifest in our physicality—in the way we stand and sit and walk, in all the things we can and cannot do. A week or two of conscientous yoga practice, and we are simultaneously confronted with the depth of our investment in a particular way of being in our bodies, and with the possibility of radical transformation. If we want the fruits of yoga, we learn that we must let go;

what's more, we learn that we can let go. We learn that there is nothing to defend, and that there never was. Pliant, supple, responsive, we become disciples of life.

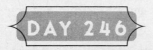

DAY 246

To make knowledge productive we will have to learn to see both the forest and the tree. We will have to learn to connect.

Peter F. Drucker

Our practice is the practice of connection. As we breathe into a posture, we bring it all together—our understanding of the problem (we do not understand who we are), our understanding of the solution (open attention in the present will reveal the truth), nonviolence, devotion, dedication without attachment. All of these principles swirl around us as we breathe into the postures of our life. Our practice is to be present so that we can make the connection between the moment we are in now and right action as it is defined by our life philosophy.

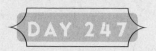

Each of you will open your heart, your actions, your wisdom,
and your conduct and look within, and you will see that every
face is your face.

His Holiness M. R. Bawa Muhaiyaddeen

As the days go by, we find that we are exploring a profound love. Yoga offers us an understanding of the world in which there is no separation, or differentiation, within the family of all beings. Our love can be all-encompassing. Growing up as an adopted child, I yearned to see someone who had my nose, my eyes. As my yoga practice deepens, I am now granted glimpses of that recognition when I look out into a forest or a crowd and allow my barriers to come down. I feel my cellular connectedness. I see my face in every face.

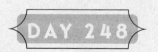

We must strive to reach that simplicity that lies
beyond sophistication.

John Gardner

I am someone who has had to work at life. Somewhere along the way, I picked up a set of rules for myself that put me in conflict with the world. I have had to unlearn those rules, and to painstakingly learn and apply a new set of rules. In the midst of all this learning and unlearning, I regularly encounter people who have no idea how complex life really is. I can spot them right away; they are the people I just can't help liking, the ones I find myself wanting to help in some way, despite the fact that they were doing just fine without me. They smile readily and have a genuine concern for the people around them. For them life is quite simple, for if you come from a place of love, the world around you will respond with love.

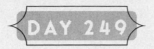

DAY 249

Out of the strain of doing, into the peace of the done.

Julia Louis Woodruff

As beginning students, most of us do not need any explanation concerning *shavasana,* or the intentional rest at the end of class. We arrive at our first yoga classes psychically drained, old before our time. To be invited to just lie back and do nothing for five minutes after an hour or so of asana feels like an amazing gift. Blessed with a beginner's mind, we simply lie back and are grateful.

As the weeks turn into months however, yoga becomes assimilated into our busy lives. We squeeze class in between our other commitments, and by the end of practice we are already planning for, worrying about, or controlling the next item on our to-do lists. Sometimes we give *shavasana* a concerted effort, more often than not, we don't. The postures are going to give us tangible results, after all; *shavasana* is just some nice spiritual ritual, like saying grace at Thanksgiving dinner, or eating matzo balls at a seder. As beginners, we understood the power of class being over, of pausing to take something in, the balance of giving and receiving. We were happy to cultivate a competence in endings, glad to lie back and let go. As more "advanced" students, we forget all that.

But we forget these lessons at our peril. *Shavasana* is called corpse pose for a reason. Death is a part of life. Avoidance of that fact is a part of the problem. Embracing the truth that things to come to an end, and showing up for that ending, is a part of the solution.

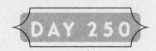

You realize that from the beginningless beginning you have been complete and whole as you are. And this supreme truth is the most difficult for us to swallow. There is nothing to be attained.

Zen master Dennis Genpo Merzel

In *shavasana* we encounter nondoing. We embrace being. We oppose the goal-driven striving of the Western world with deep stillness. This is a difficult posture for most of us. What does it mean that we have nothing to attain?

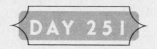

DAY 251

Observe the wonders as they occur around you. Don't claim
them. Feel the artistry moving through, and be silent.

The Prophet Muhammad

My wife and I walked down a steep hill through the jungle to a beach that
extends into Costa Rica's Manuel Antonio National Park. We walked along
the beach at sunset, as young boys on horses rode by. Later, we climbed a
mile back up the hill, straight up into the jungle. There were monkeys in
the trees, and our sweat mixed with the dust from the trail. At the top of the
trail we came to our villa. We laid our yoga mats out on the terrace overlooking the Pacific. As we practiced, the sun dipped below the ocean and it
began to rain very hard. Sheets of rain fell before us and lightning ripped
the sky. During our finishing postures, the rain slowly receded. In *shavasana*
I listened to the heavy drops fall from leaf to leaf. At the end of our practice, my wife and I sat in meditation. It was quiet after the rain. All that
could be heard was the water flowing off the leaves around us and the
sounds of the jungle coming back to life.

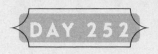

In life we must learn not only how to live, but how to die as well.

Seneca

This quote was my first introduction to the world of adult life. I was twenty-six when I read it, and although I had graduated from high school and college, had left the army and the friends I'd made during difficult years, I had not yet grasped the cycle of life, death, and rebirth that happens within a single lifetime. What Seneca taught me was that an adult lives many lives. We invest years in a moment, and then that moment passes and we must be willing to let it go, so as to be able to embrace the next moment. A study on longevity found that the common thread among those who live long is their ability to endure loss. This is the lesson of *shavasana*. We embrace a moment with all we have, and when the moment is over we step back and let go.

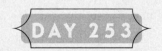
DAY 253

Be on your guard against too much cleverness.

Hermann Hesse

A while back I filled in for a friend who teaches yoga at a local gym. During the class I noticed a woman who was struggling, and I thought to myself how sad it was that she would probably never pursue yoga after the drubbing she was taking in what was clearly her first class. To my surprise, she appeared at my studio two days later to take my class. This time I felt certain that she would be too discouraged to continue. The classes at my studio are harder, longer, and about twenty degrees hotter than the class I'd taught at her gym. She stuck it out, with considerable effort, but I did not expect to see her there again. I've watched hundreds of students come and go, and this woman had all the signs of someone who would soon be going. I was certainly unprepared to see her yet again, two days later, ready for more.

Before long, she had become a regular in my 9 A.M. class. About a month later she showed up for my 7 A.M. class, on a day when she couldn't make it at nine. Arriving in the near dark on a chilly autumn morning, she demonstrated an unmistakable level of investment. After class, I asked her her name. She smiled and said, "Faith."

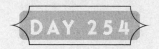

DAY 254

When you affirm big, believe big, and pray big, big things happen.

Norman Vincent Peale

We are not practicing to take the edge off. The asana are not an ancient and time-tested alternative to Valium. We are practicing asana to realize our divinity, enact it in this lifetime, and share it with all beings. By dedicating our practice to this end, we are affirming big, believing big, praying big, and allowing big things to happen.

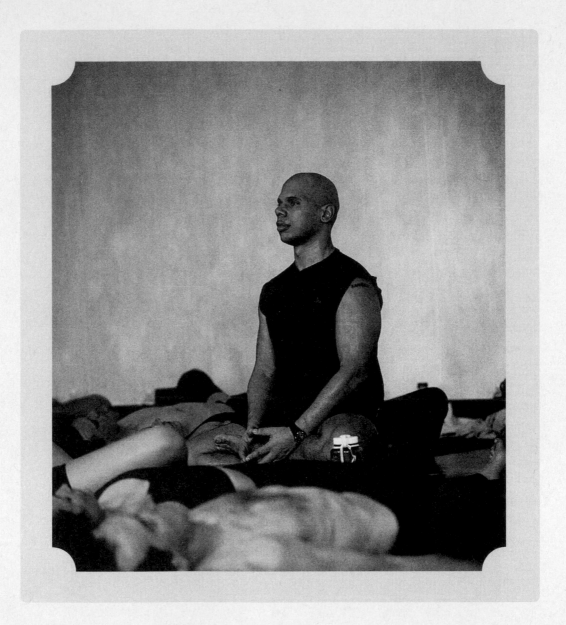

PART FOUR

PRANAYAMA

Breathing Mindfully

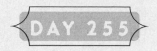

Pranayama is the regulation of the incoming and outgoing flow
of breath with retention.

Yoga Sutras

Standing at the crossroads between asana and the purely contemplative aspects of the eight-limb path, *pranayama* encompasses both the physical and the contemplative. The science of yogic breathing trains the mind in one-pointed concentration while radically improving our ability to accrue, store, regulate, and use the energy we receive from the air we breathe. Utilizing physical technique, we begin our journey into the metaphysical. The wording of the Yoga Sutras on *pranayama* is quite easy to follow. To begin, simply do what you have already been doing. Pay attention to your breath while practicing asana. Your breath should be calm and deliberate, but flowing without force or effort. Breathing in and out through the nose, let there be a pause after the inhalation, and a pause after the exhalation. If this becomes difficult, just stop and breathe freely. Begin again when it is possible to do so without difficulty. Observe the effect this measured breathing has on your physical and emotional experience. Follow the ebb and flow of your attention. *Pranayama* and asana, energy and matter.

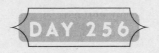

If you are in the now, you'll know how.

Baron Baptiste

The limbs of *tapas,* or action, bind us to the moment. They are actions taken or not taken in the present. The *yamas* do away with those negative actions that create remorse about the past and fear about the future. The *niyamas* take the energy freed up by the *yamas* and channel it into actions that promote health in ourselves and others. The asana simultaneously teach us to stay with the matter at hand, while deconstructing the personality flaws that induced us to hide out in our imaginations in the first place. *Pranayama* trains the mind to concentrate on one point while further refining our physical and emotional health. Consistent practice of these four limbs teaches us to live in the moment.

A simple way to get started is to focus on your breath, either in a posture, in meditation, or just while commuting to work. Note the experience you are having as you imagine your day or go over something that happened yesterday. What is your experience of yourself? Now remember or imagine a best-case scenario, in which you do a very good deed. What is your experience of yourself even in that peak, best-case imagined moment? Then return to the breath. Feel your entire body as you breathe. Listen to the sounds around you, and stay with that long enough to fully arrive in the moment. What is your experience of yourself?

This is the work of the first four limbs. It is learning to live in the moment, from the heart, in the light of our spirit. It is not about retreating from or shunning the stress and responsibilities of everyday life. Rather, it is the practice of embracing our reality with all our heart. "But, but, but . . ."

If you are in the now, you'll know how. "But, but, but . . ." If you are in the now, you'll know how. We are divine consciousness. As long as we are connected to that truth, what could possibly go wrong?

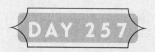

DAY 257

Enhancing the respiratory function is the surest and simplest
way to increase the adaptive capacity in the organism.

Thomas Myers

The physical benefits of *pranayama* are not esoteric. Most of us come to asana practice with restricted respiratory functioning. The muscles of respiration are often tight or weak or both. Our musculoskeletal systems have contracted to further decrease our capacity to breathe freely, and our hearts just aren't in it. Most of us simply don't care about our breath, as long as it isn't offensive. Asana practice begins the work we must do to turn this unhealthy situation around. Our entire bodies are opened up, our movements are freed, and we learn to bring our attention to the process of life flowing into and out of our bodies. *Pranayama* takes this one step further. It is the process of understanding the physiology of breathing, and the manner in which we can maximize our body's capacity to breathe.

The pages that follow will provide you with a means to begin your journey. Once you get started, seek out a teacher you like and trust, and allow him or her to guide you. The exercises in this book are simple and entirely safe; they are the same ones I was taught when I began. Much is made in some circles about *pranayama* being dangerous or too esoteric, or the province of the expert. That has not been my experience of the simple *pranayama* techniques I will teach you and have already taught to the thousands who come to my classes.

Today, spend five to ten minutes lying on your back before you practice. Close your eyes and follow your breath. Pause after the in breath, then pause after the out breath—no force, no effort. If this becomes difficult, stop, breathe freely, and when you are ready, begin again. This is enough for one day. Inhale. Pause. Exhale. Pause. Inhale. Pause. Exhale. Pause. Take this simple journey and see where it leads you.

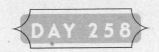

Our breath is constantly rising and falling, ebbing and flowing, entering and leaving our bodies. Full body breathing is an extraordinary symphony of both powerful and subtle movements that massage our internal organs, oscillate our joints, and alternately tone and release all the muscles in the body. It is a full participation in life.

Donna Farhi

Before your practice today, get three bed pillows. Place two on your mat and lie down on them lengthwise, with the base of the pillows just above your sacrum, or the base of your spine. This should support your spine, while lengthening it without discomfort. Your chest should be open and relaxed. Then fold the third pillow in half and place it under your head so that your chin tucks gently toward your chest. Imagine that your torso is a water glass. The base of the glass is at your hips, and the top of the glass is under your collarbones. As you inhale, the glass fills from the bottom up. As you exhale, the glass empties from the top down. Pause at the end of each inhalation and each exhalation. Remember, no force, no effort. If this becomes difficult, stop, breathe freely, and when you are ready, begin again. I often set a timer for ten or fifteen minutes so that I don't have to worry about time. But it is also nice to just allow yourself to perform this gentle *pranayama* until you feel ready to begin your asana practice. Once you begin your practice, allow the rhythm you have established with your breathing to be the rhythm of your practice.

DAY 259

The breath is an exquisite pointer to our true nature as Consciousness. The breath, like thought, is discontinuous. It comes and goes. By focusing on the pause between breaths, you open to an awareness of stillness, which lies behind and between each breath and each thought. During yoga, and in the still moments of daily life, return to this basic stillness at the end of each breath, movement, and thought.

Richard C. Miller, Ph.D.

It is said that the breath is the bridge between the body and the spirit. *Pranayama* is a practice that we experience both physically and spiritually. The moment we close our eyes and bring our attention to our breath, distinct, positive physiological effects commence. Our heart rate slows, cardiopulmonary stress is decreased, there is a decrease in metabolic activity, blood sugar and lactate levels, muscle tension, and skin conductivity. The sum total of these positive changes is an increased sense of well-being, a sense of coming home. This shift on the emotional level is accompanied by a shift in attention. We are aware that the concerns that held us so tightly just a moment before have receded. We sense a powerful presence. Richard Miller calls this presence stillness. Experience for yourself the peace of a mindful breath, enter into that stillness, and you will have a glimpse of the grandeur of the universe.

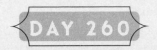

Devi: O Shiva, what is your reality? What is this wonder-filled universe? What constitutes seed? Who centers the universal wheel? What is this life beyond form pervading forms? How may we enter it fully, above space and time, names and descriptions? Let my doubts be cleared!
Shiva: Radiant one, this experience may dawn between two breaths.

Ancient Tantric text

The awareness that something happens when we bring our attention to our breath is older than recorded history and is attested to in all the world's great religions. *Pranayama,* though perhaps the oldest system, is simply one of the countless practices that have arisen to teach us to see through the veil of the distracted mind and glimpse the true nature of our existence. Our minds drift to and fro, buffeted by sensation like a boat upon stormy seas. The breath serves as an anchor, something to which we tether our minds so that we can be present for the real. What happens when you close your eyes and follow your breath? What is your truth? When you pause in a posture to feel and hear your breath, is there something there? Yoga is not meant for experts, it is meant for human beings. What is your experience when you connect to your own breath?

P R A N A Y A M A

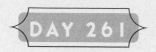

Respiration being disturbed the mind becomes disturbed. By restraining respiration, the Yogi gets steadiness of mind.

Hatha Yoga Pradipika

Over the next few days we will go on a journey across the ages and across cultures to see what has been said about the link between attention to and control of the breath and spiritual health. Here, in one of the oldest texts on hatha yoga, the branch of yoga that perfected asana practice, we are given some straightforward advice. If our breathing is chaotic, our minds and emotions will be chaotic as well. If our breathing is steady, our minds and emotions will be steady. This has been borne out in clinical studies and can be readily tested as you move through your day. Stopping in the middle of a difficult moment and bringing your attention to your breath is an excellent response. This becomes increasingly easy if you spend some time at the beginning of your day connecting to your breath.

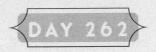

Your breath should be light, even and flowing, like a thin stream of water running through the sand. Your breath should be very quiet, so quiet that a person sitting next to you cannot hear it. Your breathing should flow gracefully, like a river, like a water snake crossing the water, and not like a chain of rugged mountains or the gallop of a horse. To master our breath is to be in control of our bodies and our minds. Each time we find ourselves depressed and find it difficult to gain control of ourselves by different means, the method of watching the breath should always be used.

Thich Nhat Hanh

Here, a present-day Buddhist teacher echoes the same ancient wisdom. Our breath, like the energy we put forth in asana, should be steady and relaxed, calm and deliberate. Over time, yoga is meant to bring us to an evenness of vision. We will come to see neither good nor bad situations, only opportunities for growth, moments in which to share and experience love. We will come to see neither good nor bad people, neither good nor bad creatures, only brothers and sisters. The early training we receive in this is to meet each posture with the same intention, each breath with the same intention. When we forget this, we are to remember and begin again.

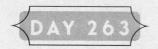

The body is the field of righteousness and also of tribulation. It
is the former when used for good and the latter when used for
bad. It is the field, and the Self is the knower thereof.
Pranayama is the bond between the two.

B. K. S. Iyengar

B. K. S. Iyengar speaks to the metaphysical side of *pranayama*. The body is
the field, the place, where it all goes down. We feel anger, fear, desire, loss,
madness, and boredom on the field of our bodies, our emotions. The self,
the witness, that which makes choices, is the knower. Ram Dass tells of a
moment when a person on LSD called him late at night. After trying unsuc-
cessfully to communicate with this individual, he told him, "I want to speak
to the person who dialed the phone." Even in the midst of a drug-induced
crisis, a part of this person knew to reach out for help, knew who to call,
and remembered his number. In our darkest moments, our true self does
not abandon us. The insight of *pranayama* is that the breath is a physiological
link between the eternal self and the field of ever-changing sensation. As
we gain control over the breath, the voice of the witness can be heard over
the din of our experience.

PART FOUR

Breathing Mindfully

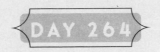
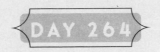 DAY 264

> The human body is a complex spiritual instrument. Ordinary
> physical breathing is not only the exchange of oxygen and carbon
> dioxide, it is the link to our light body. With every inhale-exhale
> a parallel energy flow in our light body is occurring. Bringing
> attention to the outer breath cultivates a growing awareness
> of this inner breath, harmonizes these interpenetrating
> bodies, and quiets the mind. In breath the visible and the
> invisible worlds meet.
>
> Coleman Barks and Michael Green

These writers, approaching the breath from a Sufi perspective, are in complete accordance with the views on *pranayama* held within the yogic tradition. In yogic physiology, the body is only our outermost sheath, or level of embodiment. There are seven sheaths that comprise our true body, and they coexist similarly to the three aspects of the brain. As we evolved, our brains evolved in three distinct phases. Each aspect of the brain governs different aspects of our physical, emotional, and intellectual existence while inhabiting essentially the same space. So it is with the seven sheaths of yogic physiology. The light body, as it is described in the Sufi tradition, corresponds to the breath sheath in yogic tradition. The simplest way to comprehend these visible and invisible aspects of yourself is to think of how you are affected by an emotion. Excitement, for example, is both a physical happening—affecting the dilation of our eyes, the blood flow to our extremities, our glandular exertions, and our heart and respiration rates—and an intellectual happening, an interpretation of a given situation. The intellectual happening is invisible, but our bodily reaction is readily visible. Our minds react to external stimuli: "This is a very bad thing." Our bodies react to what our minds are telling them: "Go into overdrive; this could be the big one!" At the same time, though, our witness is able to observe all of this and to send the intention of calm and deliberate breathing. The breath calms and focuses the mind and quiets our bodily reaction, harmonizing the body and mind with the intention of spirit. In this manner the breath dances within and links the different layers of our experience.

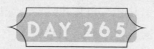

DAY 265

Meditation practice is regarded as a good and in fact excellent way to overcome warfare in the world: our own warfare as well as greater warfare.

Chogyam Trungpa Rinpoche

Meditation is the ultimate goal of *pranayama,* and in fact *pranayama* is our first step into formal meditation practice. Our work up to now has, to some extent, been external. With the *yamas* and *niyamas* each of us must work out for ourselves where to draw the line and how we want to live our daily lives. In asana the waters become clearer. There are no cultural or gender issues to be taken into consideration; either you are balancing in tree pose or you're not. In the *yamas* and the *niyamas,* and in asana, we begin to confront our demons. In *pranayama* we take a stand. If we use the opportunity to practice *pranayama* properly—that is, if we take responsibility for everything we do and do not do—we will authentically encounter our blocks to love. We will come to know the nature of our own war with reality, and we'll develop the willingness to let it go.

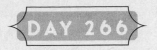

DAY 266

Conscious breathing, which is a powerful meditation in its own right, will gradually put you in touch with the body. . . . As soon as your habitual state changes from being out of the body and trapped in your mind, to being in the body and present in the Now, your physical body will feel lighter, clearer, move alive.

Eckhart Tolle

When we bring our attention to the breath, we are changing planes, moving from one level of existence to another. Our suffering is largely due to our imagined relationship to the past or to the future; the breath, however, is a doorway to the present. Not only are we gaining significant and well-documented health benefits by paying attention to our breathing, we are also consciously leaving an imagined world and entering the real. Stop reading for a moment. Sit up comfortably, close your eyes, and take ten breaths with your attention resting in the present moment, the present breath. It's powerful. It's real. It is the opportunity you've been waiting for.

PART FOUR

Breathing Mindfully

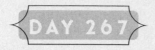

This current of the Dhikr, the remembrance of God,
is something we discover, not create. It is always
flowing in and out with the breath, like a secret tide.

Coleman Barks and Michael Green

When I was very young, I used to hide behind a corner when my class went from one building to another. I enjoyed the chaos of my interactions with my fellow first graders, but there was a magic that called to me in the quiet that I would experience when I walked, alone, back to our home room. In those few moments outdoors, I could smell the earth around me, the grass, the trees. I was alone, but not alone; this was time spent with God. Later, when I was living overseas as part of a group of men dedicated to killing other men, and sliding into an alcoholic hell, I longed for the woods of New England. There was something about the smell of pine trees and wet grass on a quiet New England afternoon that still seemed like heaven to me. Sober, I returned to New England and sought to renew my childhood connection with the earth and sky. With my oldest friend, I began to go way up into northern Maine, where we would spend weeks in a canoe, fishing on beautiful lakes, surrounded by pine trees and silence. The gratitude I felt for having survived my active addiction and for living to savor those moments with my friend in the wilderness cannot be put into words. But you will have some idea how I felt if you pause right now to breathe with your full attention. Spend a moment in silence, and open yourself to what is. Discover the secret tide, and float on it for a little while.

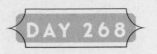

Through the practice of *pranayama* the mind
becomes arrested in a single direction.

Sri K. Pattabhi Jois

Why would we want to cultivate a mind capable of one-pointed attention? And how does that benefit us spiritually? It has been my experience that where my attention is, there I am. If I am listening to you with my undivided attention, I am with you. If my mind wanders, I'm not there either. My ability to show up for anything is predicated upon my ability to get my mind to cooperate. If we want to love anything, communicate anything, accomplish anything, we must have a mind that will go along with the plan. It is this very ability that *pranayama* practice is cultivating.

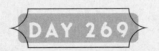

Take my yoke upon you, and learn from me; for I am gentle
and humble in heart, and you will find rest for your souls.
For my yoke is easy, and my burden is light.

Matthew 11:29–30

My *pranayama* teacher gets up in the morning and sits to meditate. If she feels like it, she will do *pranayama,* or she will simply sit. Later she will practice asana, teach asana, and study with her teacher. She has traveled around the world to learn about yoga, and she has dedicated a good portion of her house and her life to sharing yoga with others. Her practice takes up a lot of time and is a lot of work, but at sixty-four, she marries the body and the spirit of a thirty-year-old with the deep wisdom of an authentic spiritual teacher. Yoga practice does takes time and effort, but the alternative—living life without yoga or some other spiritual discipline—is harder. This is what I believe Jesus means when he says, "My yoke is easy, and my burden is light."

⟨ DAY 270 ⟩

The goal cannot be anything apart from the Self, nor can it be something gained afresh. If that were so, such a goal cannot be abiding and permanent. What appears anew will also disappear. The goal must be eternal and within. Find it within yourself.

Ramana Maharshi

Spend some time today with this statement by Ramana Maharshi before you practice *pranayama*. Then let your *pranayama* be dedicated to the truth contained in these wise words. As you follow your breath deeper and deeper into yourself, let the words echo within you. Come back to them over and over again in the days to come. "The goal must be eternal and within. Find it within yourself." Allow the energy of this statement to become intertwined with the energy of your asana practice and your *pranayama* practice. Continue to do so until it becomes a part of you, like your name.

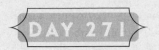

Each one of us is merely a small instrument. When you look at
the inner workings of electrical things, often you see small and
big wires, new and old, cheap and expensive, lined up. Until the
current passes through them, there will be no light. That wire is
you and me. The current is God. We have the power to let the
current pass through us, use us, produce the light of the world.
Or we can refuse to be used and allow darkness to spread.

Mother Teresa

Walking along a beach, I watched hundreds of little crabs digging tunnels
into the sand. Each crab tunnel was the equivalent of my digging a tunnel
twenty feet deep with my bare hands in thirty or forty seconds. This com-
monplace miracle was possible because it was necessary. If crabs are going to
get by in this world, they are going to have to possess that much strength,
that much life force—and so they have it. Life force is like that—ubiquitous
and inexhaustible. Nothing is impossible for those who have it. The root
word of *pranayama* is *prana,* or life force. What we call a miracle is often simply the presence of a little extra *prana.*

Prana does not differentiate between good and bad; we do. *Prana* simply
is. It infuses the mouse with the ability to run, and it infuses the hawk with
the ability to fly swiftly. It is up to each of us to make proper use of the
prana available to us. Most of us have been unconsciously minimizing the
amount of *prana* we channel into our lives because we are afraid of what we
might do with all that life force if we had it. This is why surrender to God,
or to goodness, is so important. Once we surrender, we can get on with the
business of being magnificent, trusting that we will be guided by a higher

power along the way. As we practice *pranayama,* we are learning to open up our energy channels. We're saying we are ready to be the "light of the world."

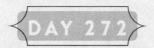

Pranayama has three movements: prolonged and fine inhalation, exhalation, and retention; all regulated with precision according to duration and place.

Yoga Sutras

These instructions, like those found in the *Hatha Yoga Pradipika,* are straightforward and easy to follow. The only mystifying reference here is to "place." Patanjali is referring to the place in the torso where the breath is retained.

In our next breathing exercise, we continue our training in "prolonged and fine inhalation, exhalation, and retention," and we introduce the concept of place.

Using your three-pillow arrangement, begin with five minutes of full breaths, including a pause after each inhalation and each exhalation. Remember, no force, no effort. Once you have settled into the breath, inhaling and exhaling for five minutes or so, exhale completely. On your next inhalation, fill the glass (your torso) only halfway up, pause, then inhale the rest of the way, filling the glass completely. Pause, then exhale completely, without a pause, until the end. Repeat the exercise, filling halfway on the inhalation, pausing, then completing the in breath. Continue this for five to ten minutes. If it becomes difficult, just stop, breathe freely, and begin again when you are ready. Ideally, at the end of this exercise, you will begin your asana practice, carrying the rhythm of your *pranayama* right into your practice. But if that is not possible, simply take a few minutes to rest in *shavasana* and continue your day, refreshed and renewed.

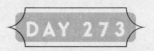

DAY 273

The wise man lets go of all results, whether good or bad,
and is focused on the action alone.

Bhagavad Gita

As I started to use what I was learning in yoga to change the way I lived, I found that my mind, my attitudes, and my beliefs were just as distorted, rigid, pain filled, and unloved as my body was. Just as it has taken me years to attain physical suppleness and well-being, so also am I finding that the process of unraveling my mental, emotional, and spiritual knots is slow work. In the face of this humbling truth, I'm learning that it is very important to take it one day at a time, to let go of results, and to focus on "the action alone."

Today, use your three-pillow arrangement and do your breathing practice for about ten minutes or so. Then pause halfway through the out breath. Once you begin the two-part out breath, stop doing the two-part in breath. Just inhale fully, pause, then exhale halfway, pause, then exhale all the way.

Now you have three distinct *pranayama* exercises to work with. Begin to explore them, and note your reactions to them. See what a good day feels like, what a bad day feels like, what difficulties you have sticking to your schedule, and why. Use your *pranayama* as a time to focus "on the action alone."

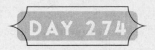
DAY 274

Taming the Bull: The whip and rope are necessary, else he might stray down some dusty road. Being well trained, he becomes naturally gentle. Then, unfettered, he obeys his master.

Kakuan

Once we begin to train our minds and our breathing in *pranayama,* we find that we need to use a significant amount of will in order to make progress. In other words, "The whip and rope are necessary." Before we know it, however, we find that something has shifted. On a given day, even the most distracted mind calms after a few minutes of practice. Next, we find that the breath we have worked so hard to regulate in *pranayama* remains regulated throughout our asana practice and as we move through the day. "Being well trained, he becomes naturally gentle." As the months become years, we find that our minds and our breath have become willing partners. "Unfettered, he obeys his master."

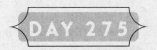
DAY 275

One must be able to let things happen.

C. G. Jung

One of the first challenges of *pranayama* is developing the ability to bring your attention to the breath without controlling it. The breath must be effortless, but we find that when we bring our attention to the breath, there is the impulse to try to control it, causing the breath to become forced. Breathing without effort is made more difficult because you are in fact slowing the breath, pausing in midbreath, pausing at the end of the in breath, pausing again at the end of the out breath. There is much to do, and there is an element of volition. Herein lies the practice. In life we also have much to do. We are parenting, working, keeping house. We are accountable to our students, employees, customers, families, and society. *Pranayama,* like the preceding three limbs of yoga, is in fact a study in subtlety in relationship, nondoing in doing, inaction in action. What we are learning as we bring our attention to our breath is the difference between intention and control. We begin *pranayama* with a clear intention, and then we let go and watch the universe respond. As we follow the breath, observing our vacillation between control and surrender, we learn to ride the breath, to experience the breath, to follow instead of lead. In our fear we believe that we must make things happen; in our practice we learn to let things happen.

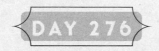

Learning that we can trust the creative energy of Life itself
enables us to relax more and more, because we know we don't
have to make things happen by force of our will.

Swami Chetanananda

I begin my asana practice with *pranayama* for two reasons. The first is that *pranayama* regulates my breathing and properly infuses my body with oxygen, so that I am physically prepared for the rigors of asana. The second is that, lying on my back with my eyes closed, watching the ocean tide of my breath, I let go. Ramana Maharshi said, "He who thinks he is the doer is also the sufferer." Lying comfortably, floating on my breath, I am reminded that I do not want to be the doer. I want to be the channel, I want to be the witness, I want to be grateful. I do not want to be the doer. That's God's job. Whenever I begin my asana practice, or anything else I do for that matter, I hold this understanding firmly in my heart and in my mind. When I let go, my whole life becomes a work of art. My actions become beneficial to myself and others.

{=+ DAY 277 +=}

According to yoga scriptures, the heart center can be opened indirectly by cultivating compassion and kindness, calmness and dispassion, or directly through the focused practice of *pranayama*, or both.

Beryl Bender Birch

The next *pranayama* technique is to be used before meditation, or on its own as a centering technique, rather than before asana. Sit up comfortably in a chair or on a cushion. Your eyes may be closed or open. Rest your left hand in your lap and bring your right hand up to your nose, the thumb resting on your right nostril, the ring finger resting on the left nostril. Close the left nostril with your finger, and exhale completely through the right nostril. Inhale through the right nostril, close the right nostril with your thumb, pause, then exhale through the left nostril. Pause, then inhale through the left nostril. Close the left nostril, pause, then exhale through the right nostril. This completes one full cycle. Continue for ten or twenty cycles, finishing by exhaling through the right nostril. If you feel dizzy, or this becomes difficult, stop, breathe freely, and when you are ready, begin again. Although it may feel awkward at first, this is not hard work. Once you have the rhythm, you'll find this to be a highly effective and centering meditative exercise. Approach it as you would anything else, steady and relaxed.

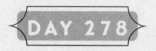

DAY 278

To identify with the ego is to identify the organism
with its history.

Alan W. Watts

The physical and mental calm that comes over us with *pranayama* practice makes it possible, often for the first time, for us to perceive the pain we are in. Rushing through our days, we feel only hints of the deep waters that swirl beneath our surface. In the stillness of practice, we dive right in. What I have found is that I have held the present a prisoner to my past. As I breathe into my body, into my life, I glimpse an alternative reality, one in which I simply am.

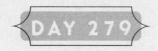
DAY 279

What is required is not a new artificial way of breathing
that lasts as long as our stunningly brief attention span, but
to return to a way of breathing that can be calm and regular,
flexible and spontaneous.

Donna Farhi

When we commit ourselves to an asana practice, we are taking our marriage vows to the breath. Unlike most marriages, though, in this one the honeymoon comes after most of the fighting is over. Over hill and dale, day in and day out, upside down, twisted like a pretzel, we call out to the breath, "Would you please help me out here? Look at me, I'm upside down! I'm twisted like a pretzel!" Over time, we find out for ourselves what Donna Farhi so eloquently articulates. We need to return, often many times in one practice, to an even, relaxed, natural breath.

As you practice asana, remain present for the work you are doing with the breath. Honor your commitment to the aptitude you are developing for *pranayama*. And as you practice *pranayama,* remain present for the aptitude you are developing in the art of breathing into a posture.

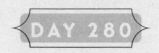

The fourth type of *pranayama* transcends the external and internal *pranayamas*, and appears effortless and non-deliberate.

Yoga Sutras

For many of us, the first experience we have with this sort of transcendent breathing comes in asana. I have also experienced it while training for marathons. It is the moment when concentration gives way to meditation. Initially we are focused on the technique. The mind becomes centered through concentration. We often stay right here at this level, moving in and out of distraction, moving in and out of concentration. If our concentration quiets us enough, though, something powerful happens. Where until now we have sought out experience, suddenly experience seeks us out instead. We cross a threshold, and meditation overtakes us. Like nightfall in a forest, one moment there is a blue-gray light; the next moment we are in darkness. In meditation, effort ceases and we are no longer the doer. Our breathing carries on without our volition, drawing us deeper into the moment with each breath. As our minds become still, we become the calm forest pool, inaction in action. This is not a mountain to climb or a grade to get. It is a place within you that you are already experiencing. Your practice merely opens the door so that you can return to this sacred place.

Those who really want to be yogis must give up, once and for all,
this nibbling at things. Take up one idea; make that one idea
your life. Think of it, dream of it, live on that idea. Let the
brain, muscles, nerves, every part of your body, be full of that
idea, and just leave other ideas alone.

Swami Vivekananda

My one idea is expressed by the word "God." I would prefer that it were "Gaia" or "Great Spirit," because they seem more inclusive, but when the Great Spirit touched me, "God" was the only word I knew, and it has stuck. Initially, God meant not drinking and helping other alcoholics get well. Working with teenage addicts, I experienced moments of human connection almost too beautiful to put into words. It was as though I was able to go back in time and to help the suffering young person I had been. Over time, I began drawing fewer lines around myself and who I would help. I have worked with the urban homeless and the rural poor, young rich kids and not so young rich kids. As I expanded my embrace and my notion of who I could help, my one idea expanded as well. Now I include myself and my family among those I can cheer on. Today, I look out across my deck in Costa Rica and watch monkeys move through the trees like schools of fish, like herds of antelope, like flocks of birds, like groups of children, and I see the underlying oneness. Like every other posture, my one idea began in doing and has become surrender.

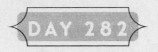

Pranayama removes the veil covering the light of knowledge
and heralds the dawn of wisdom.

Yoga Sutras

Pranayama is a turning point in our practice. Our attention has gradually been drawn inward. From the external practices of the *yamas* and *niyamas* to the body-centered practice of asana, we have progressed to the internal world of *pranayama*. In *pranayama* we begin to develop the skills that will carry us the rest of the way home—the turning of the mind inward, concentration, and meditation. Lying on the floor, practicing *pranayama* exercises, we perceive both the turbulence of our minds and the eternal stillness underneath. As we revisit this stillness day after day, we gradually become aware of an alternative to the futility of our materialist strivings. In the Bible it says that we seek but do not find. In *pranayama* we learn that this is true only if we are looking outside ourselves for what is already within. *Pranayama* confirms the central message of yoga—that we have already arrived, that we are already home, that we must simply wake up from the dream that this is not so. Wake up, live fully, be grateful, and share what you have found.

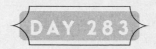

Peace is impossible to those who look on war. Peace is
inevitable to those who offer peace. How easily, then,
is your judgment of the world escaped. It is not the world
that makes peace seem impossible. It is the world you see
that is impossible.

A Course in Miracles

One of the fundamental teachings of yoga is that if you encounter a person who is established in nonviolence, you will give up violence in that person's presence. We each have within us the ability to bring an end to violence. Which is to say that the violence in our midst is our responsibility. Nation after nation does violence to another, and peace seems ever more elusive. We meet violence with more violence, and then our leaders profess shock and outrage when others do not give up their violence toward us.

Our yoga practice is a nonviolent one. Each aspect of this path teaches us *ahimsa,* or nonharming, in our dealings with ourselves and others. *Pranayama* is a profound step in this transformation. We are intentionally bringing peace to the waters of our minds. This peace, like a ripple moving across the surface of a pond, travels through us and out into the family of all beings.

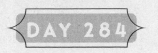

We were brainwashed.

Marianne Williamson

My mother, bless her heart, had an enormous impact on how I came to see the world. I would burst through the door and say, "It would make my heart sing if I could do X." She would respond with something like, "Oh dear, I recently read that a person was killed doing X," or, "I don't think you can do X, and only bad people do X anyway." It did not matter what X was; my mother had recently heard that someone had been killed doing it. Eventually I grew up and left home, but I continued to run my new ideas by my mom, with the same results. After thousands of squashed dreams, years of spiritual work, and countless hours on the mat, it finally dawned on me that I would be better off if I stopped trying my ideas out on my mother. While this has been effective in reducing the amount of negative feedback I receive in any given month, it has not entirely solved the problem. My mother lives on, her voice embedded in my habitual thought patterns, my habitual responses to my own ideas, passions, and abilities.

Of course, not everyone was brought up by my mother. Some of my friends feel compelled to prove themselves in business before they can give themselves permission to become writers; others can't get married because their mothers were abandoned by their fathers; some can't get divorced because their fathers stuck by their mothers. Yoga teachers often tell students that our bodies are a walking autobiography, in order to draw attention to the ways in which our bodies mirror our choices. But this is only half the story. We come to our mats as the sum total of all the beliefs we have ever encountered, absorbed, rejected, or lived. Our imaginations are like swollen rivers, flooded with the falsehoods of the ages as they have been passed on to us across the generations. Who we are, who everyone else is, and what we can be—all are defined by this river, which is not of our making.

Either we can continue to bob along on the river of our imagination or we can make our way to the shore, observe the river for a while, and then just walk away. The process of coming onto the shore is what the limbs of *tapas* are all about. There is another reality, a light that resides within us all. The actions taken and not taken in the *yamas,* the *niyamas,* the asana, and *pranayama* remove that which is blocking the light. They bring us up onto the shore and give us the strength to walk away from the river. The limbs that follow concern what happens next. For today, allow your practice to deliver you from your imagination and into the light.

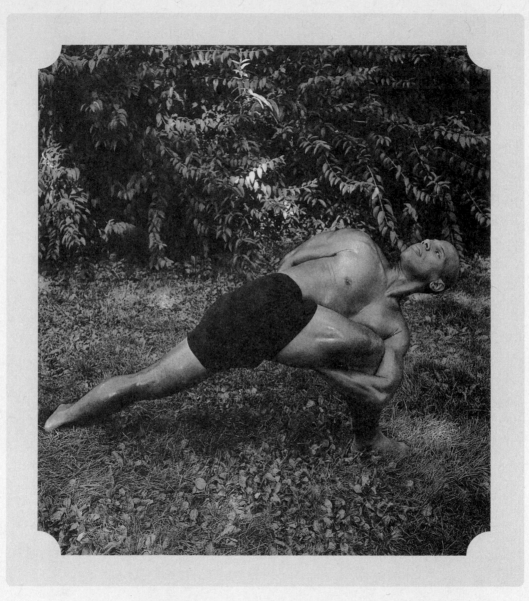

PART FIVE

PRATYAHARA

Turning Inward

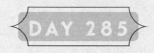

> Better than any ritual is the worship achieved through wisdom;
> wisdom is the final goal of every action.
>
> Bhagavad Gita

The second stage of the yoga path is the limbs of *svadhyaya,* or self-study. They are *pratyahara* and *dharana,* which mean turning inward and concentration. Having laid a foundation of equanimity and health with the limbs of *tapas,* or spirituality in action, we now embark on a journey of self-discovery. By and large the limbs of *tapas* are devoted to separating the true from the false, the real from the unreal. Physically, mentally, emotionally, and spiritually, *tapas* is the process of cleaning house. The limbs of *svadhyaya* are a time of turning inward and focusing upon the insights made in *tapas.*

Pratyahara is a fascinating moment in this process—the juncture at which we go from distraction to direction. This is a turning point, an intersection of two planes of existence. My favorite example of *pratyahara* in daily life is the first day or two of vacation. You have already done the work, performed your *tapas.* You have cleared the time, made the arrangements, paid your bills, farmed the dog out to your in-laws, survived the travel ordeal, and now you are finally here. Or are you? My experience of the first day or so of a vacation is the gradual process of letting go of my life at home and embracing the entirely new world of vacation. Initially, I am still absorbed by some final interaction back home, some final detail. I am usually tired and distracted. Then, gradually, I shift focus. I begin to relax into the moment. This is the process of *pratyahara*—but instead of turning our attention toward a vacation, we turn our attention inward, toward the light.

Dharana is much simpler to understand. It is holding one's attention on the light. *Dharana* is the development and utilization of our powers of concentration. *Pratyahara* and *dharana* together make possible the acquisition of wisdom. Having let go of distraction and turned a focused mind inward, we can begin to truly plumb the depths of our souls. We connect to our truth, to our true selves. In my own life, this was the point at which I began to live from my intuition. I began to cultivate and honor my own intuitive powers. I began to listen to the promptings of my heart. I began to value stillness and silence. My time on the mat went to a deeper place.

We can start where we are, by simply becoming aware of the process by which we arrive somewhere. Note the moment, the point, where your experience departs from resistance and moves into understanding. Begin to witness how it is you gain wisdom from your actions.

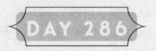

DAY 286

Withdrawing the senses, mind, and consciousness from contact with external objects, and then drawing them inwards towards the seer, is *pratyahara*.

Yoga Sutras

In the last four limbs of yoga, we leave physical technique behind and embrace an entirely internal practice. *Pratyahara* is the decision to turn inward, to let go of drama. It is the choice to release our grip on the external world and all our attempts to control it, in order to focus our minds entirely on the internal. In *pranayama* we stood astride two worlds, breathing with one foot firmly planted in physical sensation and technique, and the other planted in the internal world of concentration and meditation. *Pratyahara* is the moment when the intrepid explorers leave their boats on the shore and head inland. For today, simply bring this practice into focus. Begin with your *asana* practice, and note the edge here. At what point do you draw your boat onto the shore and head inland? What reservations do you have about doing this? What resistance do you have to letting go of the past and the future? Then observe this process of turning inward as it is played out in your daily interactions. Pay attention to where you go, where your attention is placed, as you honor your commitments to your work, your relationships, yourself. This is not meant to be hard work. Approach *pratyahara* as you would any other posture—steady and relaxed, breath flowing freely.

{ DAY 287 }

When I was a child, I spoke like a child, I thought like
a child, I reasoned like a child; when I became a man,
I gave up childish ways.

1 Corinthians 13:11

As we grow older we come to understand that we can remain enmeshed in pain masked as pleasure, or we can decide to leave the pain behind and develop new ways of moving through the world. I think of the decision to stop hurting ourselves as *pratyahara*. It is a renunciation of pain. The first four limbs of yoga are the *abhyasa,* or practice, limbs. *Pratyahara* is the beginning of the limbs of *vairagya,* or renunciation. Our practice makes clear the futility of many of our choices. *Pratyahara* and the limbs that follow are our response to that futility. We acknowledge that we were children and did not know any better. We did the best we could with what we had. But the past is over now, and it is time to put away childish things.

There is a pretty Indian fable to the effect that if it rains when the star Svati is in ascendance, and a drop of rain falls into an oyster, that drop becomes a pearl. The oysters know this, so they come to the surface when the star appears, and wait to catch the precious raindrops. When the drops fall into them, quickly the oysters close their shells and dive down to the bottom of the sea, there patiently to develop the raindrops into pearls. You should be like that. First hear, then understand, and then, leaving all distractions, shut your minds to outside influences and devote yourselves to developing the truth within you.

Swami Vivekananda

When I began working on this book, I imagined that I would teach and write at the same time. But as I got more deeply into the writing, I struggled with this plan. I asked my friend, yoga teacher and writer Beryl Bender Birch, how she managed to write her books, and she told me that she takes a couple of months away from her teaching each time she embarks on a new book. Eventually, my wife and I packed up the car and went to stay in the country. It was quiet there. I could write in the morning, then spend the afternoons out on the country trails. Some days I would walk in the hills or in the forest. Other days I would sit down in the valley by the river. One evening, we watched as hundreds of small fish leaped out of the rushing water, flashing silver like fireworks against a darkening sky. Slowly, like a pearl forming in an oyster deep in the ocean, this book took shape, as I wrote in the mornings and wandered in the afternoons.

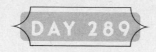

Happiness exists perennially within you. It is your normal state.
You have not to seek it. You will necessarily be happy if you get
rid of the obstacles called pain, which are in the modes of mind.
Happiness is not a secondary thing, but pain is, and these
painful things are obstacles to be got rid of. When they have
stopped, you must be happy.

Annie Besant

Nondoing is the key to happiness. To become happy, we simply have to stop making ourselves unhappy. Many of us don't believe it could be so simple. We are compelled to act out in ways that cause pain to ourselves and others. We act the way we do, we believe, because we are so unhappy. What we fail to see is that we are so unhappy because of our behavior. Aristotle wrote, "What we have the power to do, we have the power not to do." But many of us don't believe this. We have our scripts for life and we adhere to them unquestioningly. "I cannot forgive So-and-so," we tell ourselves, even if that means we will be trapped in an unhealthy relationship with this person that extends beyond the grave. Another popular script says, "I am a person who does not make mistakes, therefore I cannot say I am sorry." Yet another reads, "In my family we are not like that, and we do not do this." There are as many scripts as stars in the sky, and none of them are true unless we make them true. We are not practicing yoga to take the edge off, or to loosen up, or to get in shape. We practice yoga to become free. *Pratyahara* is about becoming free.

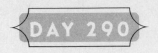

Liberty, when it begins to take root, is a plant of rapid growth.

George Washington

Letting go of our pain is not an overnight affair, but the process quickly gains momentum. It's a little like water moving through a hole in a dam. First there is just a trickle, then a small flow, then before you know it, there is a torrent. The most miraculous part of this process is in the trickle stage. This is when you see the dramatic courage, the thrilling movement and change. It is the addict's first few months of sobriety, the battered woman leaving home for good, the forty-something businessperson leaving a job and going to medical school. It's picking up the pieces after a great loss. It's trying again after a bitter failure. This is the time when you find out who your friends are and what a friend really is. Later, once the flow has become established, the work changes. Now the challenge is in staying green and fresh, remaining established in beginner's mind. *Pratyahara* is right down there at ground zero, in the field where heroes are made. It is our first steps into the light. The remaining limbs on the eight-limb path are about maintenance and growth. *Pratyahara* is about beginnings.

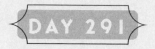

> I never lose the opportunity of urging a practical beginning,
> however small, for it is wonderful how often the mustard seed
> germinates and roots itself.
>
> Florence Nightingale

At the heart of *pratyahara* is the notion that we are already there. We are already in heaven, and heaven exists in us, right now. We must simply stop reinforcing the fear that this is not so. And so, with *pratyahara,* we begin the practice of meditation, the practice of stopping. Our first moments in meditation are a lot like slamming on the brakes in a car. All sorts of things keep moving, even though the car isn't. It takes the mind a while to figure out that we are no longer moving and that we are serious about being still. A tussle then ensues as to who will be in charge of the time spent in meditation—the restless mind, or the one who has decided to sit. This tussle is the domain of *pratyahara*. Just as there is yoga on the mat and off the mat, there is *pratyahara* on the cushion and off the cushion. On the cushion, *pratyahara* is the process of letting go of distraction. It is the twilight place between everyday consciousness and singular, pointed concentration.

For today, make a practical beginning. Set a timer for ten or fifteen minutes, and then settle yourself, sitting comfortably upright, in a chair or on a cushion. Either you can count breaths from one to ten, then from ten to one, or you can simply follow your breath as it moves in and out of your body. Use the skills you have developed in your asana and *pranayama* practice to settle your mind and body. In the quiet space of this time, become aware of the inward movement of *pratyahara*. It is a movement away from energy-draining distraction toward energy-building concentration.

And this our life exempt from public haunt,
Finds tongues in trees, books in the running brooks,
Sermons in stones, and good in everything.

William Shakespeare

Deepak Chopra has written that the ideal amount of meditation is a half hour in the morning and a half hour at night. I have done this at different times in my life, but most of the time I'm not able to manage it. What I have done is "a little a lot" rather than "a lot a little." If you can develop the habit of meditating for just fifteen minutes in the morning, you will be well on your way. When my worklife has been most stressful, taking even fifteen minutes has been a challenge, and yet that is when meditation has proved to be indispensable. When my work has required me to be highly creative over long periods of time, meditation has been even more important. We live our lives hovering above the source, just out of reach of the ocean of wisdom that has inspired artists and scholars, leaders and parents over the ages. Meditation takes us right into this ocean. *Pratyahara,* the process of turning inward, is our walk across the beach and our will to jump in. My experience of even fifteen minutes a day of meditation is as Shakespeare describes it. Whether or not I feel as though I had a good meditation, the world just opens up before me. My heart and my mind become calm, and in that calm I become a channel of grace.

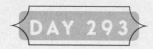

John F. Kennedy . . . meant something to this country while he was alive. More significant, however, is what we do with what is left, with what has been started. It was his conviction, like Plato's, that the definition of citizenship in a democracy is participation in government and that, as Francis Bacon wrote, it is "left only to God and to the angels to be lookers on."

Robert F. Kennedy

Sloth would have us be spectators in our own lives. On the mat we can move through sloth fairly easily by focusing on the posture at hand. The energy released by our practice dissipates sloth so readily that by the end of yoga class most of us have forgotten all the resistance we were contending with at the beginning. In meditation, however, sloth is a more formidable foe. I go for a walk or take a shower before I meditate in the morning, so that I will be wide awake. I avoid meditating soon after I have eaten, and I don't try to meditate late at night. Even so, I encounter sloth in meditation. Often it's a result of fear. Some area of my life is out of balance and I'm afraid. Fear sets me up, then sloth comes in for the kill: "I don't have to practice today." "I don't have to follow through with what I've set out to do." "I am too tired to participate in my own life today." It's important for me to see sloth as a symptom of unresolved issues in my life. Sloth rears its head when I'm dealing with situations I wish to avoid and fears that I am unwilling to confront. All of this robs me of the sort of agency in my own life that the Kennedy brothers so beautifully modeled in public life. *Pratyahara* is the recognition that we are not meant to be onlookers in our own lives, but full participants, no matter what.

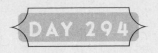

DAY 294

Being still has been very liberating. I am better able
to unhook, be present, not react, breathe. And maybe
tomorrow I'll forget, but maybe I won't.

Alyssa S., yoga student

It is important not to get too wrapped up in doing it right. As the Nike ad says, just do it. Sit comfortably, being quiet, for ten or fifteen minutes a day. That's it. Let your meditation practice build on its own momentum. Don't cheat it; treat it with respect and don't worry about it. If you wish to, find a meditation center. But a cushion on the bedroom floor is a fine place to start. Go on meditation retreats if you can, and once there, remember to take what you need and leave the rest. Meditation teachers and meditators are just human beings trying to get better. Their teachings and their behaviors are not your problem. The only thing you need to do is bring your own butt to your own meditation cushion today, tomorrow, and the day after that.

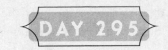

DAY 295

Be your breath, ah, smile, hey, and relax, ho,
and remember this, you can't miss.

Rick Fields

One of the first obstacles we encounter when we begin meditation practice is doubt. We believe that we are constitutionally incapable of meditating.

We are not sitting right, our back hurts, our mind is racing, this is point-less . . . Oh, forget it! Meditation is not rocket science. You have been doing a form of it in asana and *pranayama* already. This is simply a more effortless form of yoga than you are used to. Let go. "Be your breath, ah, smile, hey, and relax, ho, and remember this, you can't miss."

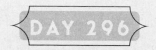

How do you know you are confronting a classic "hindrance" on your spiritual path? Just ask yourself: am I losing my sense of balance, my sense of priorities, and my sense of what's really important? Am I being carried away by temporary reactions, by destructive emotions? That's what challenges do; they obstruct your insight and prevent you from seeing things as they really are. They stand between you and the calm clear awareness of the enlightened mind.

Lama Surya Das

The Buddha listed five hindrances, or challenges, on the spiritual path. And we encounter all of them in the stillness of meditation. They are craving, ill will, sloth and torpor, restlessness, and doubt. We've just talked about doubt. But once we get past the phantom of doubt and have begun a regular practice, we encounter all the rest of the challenges. The five hindrances are unlike the five afflictions of yoga in that they are not outlining humanity's essential predicament; rather, they are are merely defining the negative habits of the mind that are a result of that predicament. These habits of mind are alive and well amidst the distractions of everyday life. Coming to a complete stop in meditation is like turning on a light in a room full of ants.

All of a sudden our craving, our restlessness, our doubts, resentments, and sloth are revealed to us in the bright light of a mind without its normal distractions. It is the very effectiveness of meditation, in its ability to reveal to us the habitual pathways of our minds, that convinces many of us that meditation isn't working. Understanding that these habits are alive in our lives and that they are not who we are is the first step in the process called *pratyahara*.

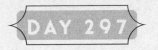

DAY 297

It's not that life is so comfortable from my point of view, it's just that when one is willing to let life in and let life out, it's more comfortable than when one is in resistance to life all the time.

Patricia Townsend, yoga teacher

Craving is one of the classic Buddhist hindrances on the spiritual path. It has so many faces that one of my own greatest cravings is for there to be an end to craving. This morning I spent a half hour reading about the first bombings of Afghanistan. I then spent another thirty minutes reading tributes to individuals who died on September 11—a father who had a quick appointment on the ninety-sixth floor, brothers who worked on the 104th and 105th floors, a young woman who had just graduated from college and was heading for her first business trip to the West Coast. By the end of this, I did not feel like writing. I didn't feel like doing anything. I was scared and sad. I craved another life, another situation. I did not want to embrace my life. But I put one foot in front of another. I was motivated in part by the support I'm getting from my wife and my editors as I write these pages. I got myself oriented, read over my last few essays, and began the process of writing today's essay. As I practiced the familiar action steps of writing, my craving for relief, my desire not to be who I am receded. I began to have the feeling that I have something to offer. As I took actions that give meaning to my life, my resistance to life lessened. When we are in craving, we are withdrawing from our life; our practice is a pathway back.

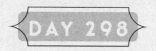

DAY 298

Thoughts are energy, and you can make your world
or break your world by your thinking.

Susan Taylor

Every so often an experienced yoga student comes to my class for the first time and has a really bad time of it. Despite the fact that her body has been trained, her mind has remained untamed. Usually within the first few minutes, the class becomes something that she opposes. As the class progresses, her resentment builds, until I can almost see what's running through her mind: "This is just plain wrong. These people are just not doing this right, and by God it makes me angry!" She is in hell. She is having an attack of what the Buddha called ill will. It is in the nature of ill will to be extroverted. The problem is out there, not in here. Ill will is pervasive. We experience it everywhere, nearly all of the time, and it usually makes no sense. I recently felt ill will toward my wife because she wanted to be listened to when I wanted to be listened to, too. How could she be so selfish? The problem isn't that we experience feelings of ill will, the problem is that we allow ourselves to go with them. Asana practice and meditation are excellent places to address our tendency to run with ill will. In meditation, and later as you move through your day, name ill will as it comes up. Observe it arise, then name it; say to yourself, "Ill will." Begin to see how ill will has the power to define the world you live in, or not, depending on your reaction to it.

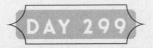

DAY 299

> The next time you communicate with anyone, you can put aside
> your own autobiography and genuinely seek to understand. . . .
> Don't push; be patient; be respectful. People don't have to
> open up verbally before you can empathize. You can empathize
> all the time with your behavior. You can be discerning, sensitive,
> and aware, and you can live outside your autobiography.
>
> Stephen R. Covey

The final Buddhist hindrance to practice is restlessness. Restlessness needs no explanation, but I will give it one anyway. Restlessness is our inability to sit with what is. Stephen Covey identifies restlessness as one of the main blocks to communication and connection with others. Restlessness hovers about everything we do; it is the offspring of *abhinivesa,* our fear of death. It is also, as Covey points out, an offspring of all the fears we have learned, a product of our autobiography. In asana and meditation we are training ourselves to embody the moment. In so doing, we are embracing all of the moment, and part of this is about accepting the moment's passing. We are learning not to begrudge the need for things to end. Restlessness is a manifestation of our resistance to this. We do not want to relinquish control. As we slip into stillness, and into the ego death that comes with stillness, we start to bob and weave. Suddenly we have to fix our hair, adjust our clothes, scratch an itch, cough, sneeze, or sigh. Our minds travel off into an imagined past or future, we make plans for events that will never come to pass, we make a grocery list for dinner. Then we remember—stillness!—and we begin again. Instead of fighting your restlessness, just name it. Acknowledge it as it arises. You can do this in meditation, on the mat, or the next time you talk with someone. Put aside your autobiography and allow yourself to simply be present with what is.

DAY 300

> Your mind blocks the free flow of life by saying, "This is how things must and should be." Letting go releases you from this insistent grip, and when you let go, new forms of reality can enter.
>
> Deepak Chopra

The practice of *pratyahara* entails examining one's attachments. "Do those amazing apple pancakes really make me feel better?" "What happens when I play the big shot and open my mouth when I shouldn't?" "Would it be so horrible if X happens, and even if it is that horrible, is it worth the sacrifice I am making to avoid it?" At the beginning of this book, I wrote about fear of death being an obstacle to happiness. Maybe you rolled your eyes. But what is driving our attachment? Is life linear? Are we given a finite number of things to enjoy? When we lose one of those things, are we forever diminished? Does death steal away all that we have? And what about *having?* Can we really own or lose anything? Do we own the breath we breathe, the force that keeps our heart beating? What is it that death steals away, anyway? If we can attain even a "Who knows?" attitude, things will start to ease up. Letting go is the opposite of fearing death; it is trusting life. When we let go of something, our hand opens and we are able to receive.

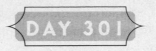

DAY 301

> It is never too late for any of us to look at our minds. We can always sit down and allow the space for anything to arise. Sometimes we have a shocking experience of ourselves. Sometimes we try to hide. Sometimes we have a surprising experience of ourselves. Often we get carried away. Without judging, without buying into our likes and dislikes, we can always encourage ourselves to just be here again and again and again.
>
> Pema Chodron

At the very heart of our practice we need one thing: a mature willingness to no longer be in pain. This willingness is *pratyahara*. It comes from experience, it comes from the decision to learn from experience, it comes from acknowledging that we are of God but not God, and it comes from the belief that we can be free. The action we must take contains a paradox. We must acknowledge powerlessness as our essential condition—after all, we do not even control the beating of our own hearts—and yet, at the same time, we must acknowledge our absolute responsibility for our actions. Adrift on a sea not of our making, we must acknowledge that we are defined by the choices that we make. Our meditation practice teaches us to bear witness to who we are and who we might become.

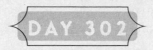

Simple, clear purpose and principles give rise
to complex and intelligent behavior.

Dee Hock

Keep it simple. *Pratyahara* is all about action. When you come to your meditation cushion or your yoga mat, you have made a decision to show up. *Pratyahara* is showing up; it's letting go of the past and the future and being here now; it's letting grace happen. Off the cushion, off the mat, it is being clear in your intention to grow. Whenever I teach a yoga class, I spend the entire class in the presence of decision. I can either play it safe, be cool, and not grow, or I can take a risk, show up, and grow. Taking a risk implies courage, but the pain of acting out cowardice is even greater than the discomfort that comes with a risk. Keeping it simple is knowing this, accepting this, and acting on it.

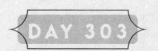

There is a secret one inside us; the planets like
galaxies pass through his hands like beads.

Kabir

All of the great religions, teachings, mystics, and sages describe a secret one, a lotus flower at our center. The world abounds with evidence of this inner being. There is no end to the art, music, humor, and literature sprung from this deep well of creativity. Over and over again, artists and writers, attempting to explain the source of their creations, refer to some mysterious inner guide. *Pratyahara* is the moment in yoga when we decide to let our answers come from within. In asana we embody inspiration, in meditation we allow inspiration, in prayer we commune with inspiration. Twelve-step programs use the electric phrase "having made the decision to turn our will and our lives over to the care of God." *Pratyahara* is having made the decision.

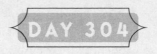

My grace is sufficient for you.

Jesus

Pratyahara is a leap of faith. In meditation, our task is fairly simple. Our minds are wedded to the habit of distraction, and we train them to let go of this habit. We move from distraction to direction. In life, it is a lot scarier. We have the habit of doing what our family, culture, friends, and spouse think is right, and we have to train ourselves, instead, to listen to our own heart. Even harder is letting go of our habit of acting out of fear. Fortunately, our practice clears things up. We gain an understanding of where we are and where we want to go. Eventually, though, we stand at the edge of the abyss. "I know that I must do X, but what if I fall?" Each of us must face those moments alone and find out for himself. What I have witnessed, experienced myself, and learned from the experiences of others through the ages is that the love that wished you into existence will never let you down.

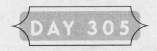

The boisterous sea of liberty is never without a wave.

Thomas Jefferson

And so we are embarking on the boisterous sea of liberty—boisterous, because *pratyahara* is enacted at every level of our existence. It is the smallest and simplest decision; it is the most momentous as well. We are presented with opportunities to walk away from our self-inflicted pain at all hours of the day and night, and with each new liberty comes a new awareness, a new challenge. While I've been writing this book, I have also been in a quiet war with the man who takes care of my building. He does not like my dog. Even as I've written in these pages about love, I've found it just too hard to forgive this man. We have resented each other now for over two years. As my daily writing has seeped deeper into my consciousness, my enthusiasm for this war has waned. In the face of dire provocation, I have exercised restraint. Recently I said hello to this man and smiled genuinely. Later, he opened the door for me as I came in with my dog.

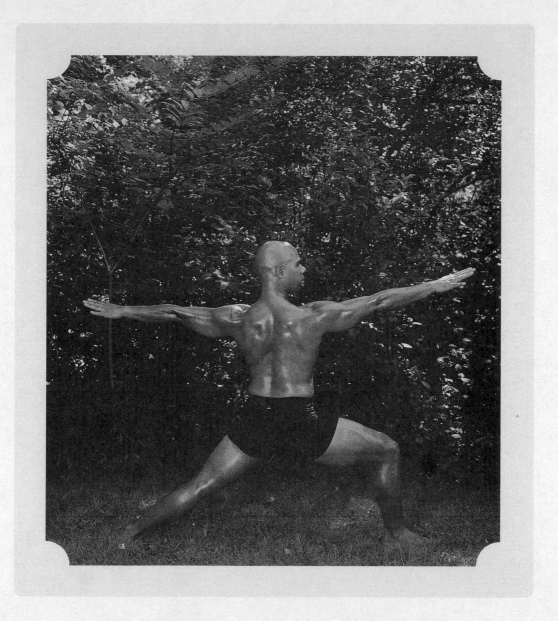

PART SIX

DHARANA

Concentration

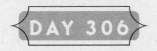

Fixing the consciousness at one point or region is concentration.

B. K. S. Iyengar

The next limb on the eight-limb path is *dharana,* or concentration. We learn to bring our attention to one point, and we train our minds to stay there. The point of concentration can be external, as in asana, or it can be internal, as in meditation. On the mat we experience *dharana* quite often, during those moments when we lose track of time, when our minds become so absorbed in the physical experience of a posture that we are no longer connected to everyday concerns. In *dharana,* the past and the future have dissolved and we are simply existing in the now. I experience *dharana* in every class I teach, and that is how I knew that teaching yoga was a healing path for me. Most of us are fortunate enough to have found activities that draw forth this deep concentration. When we are doing something we truly love, we cannot help but give ourselves to it wholeheartedly. *Dharana,* therefore, is a by-product of love. In the clarity of a focused mind, we find that timeless place where we connect to spirit. In this sense, *dharana* is our pathway to spirit.

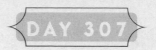

D H A R A N A

You may ask yourself what that state would be in which there is no mind, no knowledge. What we call knowledge is a lower state than one beyond knowledge. You must always bear in mind that extremes look very much alike. If a very low vibration of ether is taken as darkness, and an intermediate state as light, a very high vibration will be darkness again. Similarly, ignorance is the lowest state, knowledge is the middle state, and beyond knowledge is the highest state; the two extremes seem the same. Knowledge itself is a manufactured something, a combination; it is not Reality.

Swami Vivekananda

In baseball, pitchers are told, "Throw the ball, don't aim it." This is a good example of the difference between knowledge and the knowing that is beyond knowledge. To aim the ball is to come from a place of knowledge, of trying to control events. To throw the ball is to let go into the flow of the moment, to trust events and your place in them. To aim the ball is to affirm your separateness; to throw the ball is to affirm your connectedness. In aiming there is much mental chatter; in throwing there is no sound; there does not need to be. The regularity of asana and meditation practice provides us with the chance to see both forms of activity for what they are. We can think about a posture or we can embody it fully, without reservation. We can sit in meditation at war with ourselves, trying to stay with the breath, or we can surrender and soften into stillness. *Dharana* is throwing the ball. It is the quiet that occurs when we flow into a posture or let go into meditation. It is the mind pouring itself like water into a moment. It is the stillness that is beyond knowledge.

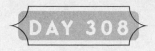

DAY 308

Now if you want to be saved you must be guided
to think beyond words.

Roy Masters

Dharana is not something we *do,* it is something that happens. It is the result of surrendering to love. In the gladness of love, we let go of our resistance to life. The present moment becomes acceptable and we are overtaken by the real. We experience this as *dharana.* The words we use to describe it are "deep concentration" or "flow," but in fact what we are experiencing is deep connection. The elite baseball player's mind opens so fully that he can perceive and connect with a baseball traveling ninety-five miles per hour. In this place of deep connection, he follows the movements, the subtlest fluctuations of the ball, and responds to them intuitively—all of the millions of movements that must be orchestrated in order for him to hit that ball are fully understood and flawlessly executed in a timeless instant. There is a knowing that is beyond words, a moment that is beyond time.

In the deep connection that is *dharana,* we are alive in a fashion that bears only a slight resemblance to ordinary life. We have applied ourselves to something we love—be it gardening, race car driving, parenting, meditation, or asana practice—and we have withstood the rigors of love. In our fidelity we have broken through our fear and found ourselves in a state of deep connection. Love draws us deep into itself; deep into a place beyond space and time, fear and doubt, words and failure. Each time we are drawn into this place, we emerge forever changed. The qualities of this place have become more real to us, more accessible. We find that we are guided by a thinking that is beyond words.

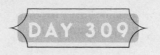

When our perceptions are no longer dressed up or boxed in by
our endless list of ideas, we can understand what is meant by
"Seeing things as they are." When we are very, very still, in the
way that meditation allows us to be, we can find the space to let
everything be as it is. It is from that space that you will find the
room you need to see who you are and how you fit in the world.

Angel Kyodo Williams

This morning I took the 7 A.M. class at my studio. Afterward, I fell into
conversation with a student I've known by sight for a couple of years but
have never had a chance to talk with at any length. In the relaxed atmos-
phere immediately after class, we discussed our passion for asana practice.
He told me that he's had a spiritual practice for many years, the basis of
which is Bible study, and that he finds that his yoga practice enriches his
connection to God. Walking out into the cool orange, blue, and brown of
an early fall morning, he said, "God resides in stillness, a stillness which is in
my heart. And yoga reconnects me to that stillness."

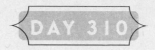

The world is evolving from imperfection towards perfection;
it needs all love and sympathy; great tenderness and
watchfulness is required from each one of us.

Hazrat Inayat Khan

The asana classes I teach, and this book as well, are intended to be of use to the householder. I think of a householder as an individual who has not chosen to take monastic vows but has instead decided to live in the flow of mainstream society, probably juggling a family and a career. Householders are members of the class of people who perform the difficult functions that make our civilization possible. They are the teachers, police officers, doctors, lawyers, soldiers, construction workers, scientists, and parents—some of the people we most admire, people who have embraced their roles wholeheartedly and have turned their daily work into an expression of love. Householders care for the young and care for the old. They work hard, and their bodies and minds must be able to withstand the rigors of service. Asana practice and meditation are ideally suited for sustaining the householder as he or she carries the burdens of adulthood.

Hazrat Inayat Khan describes the most important responsibilities of a householder—the requirement that we move through the world as channels for love and sympathy, conducting ourselves with great tenderness and watchfulness. The asana develop our ability to act with great tenderness and watchfulness. When this ability becomes pronounced, we call it *dharana,* or the opposite of fear. To care for our world, to give loving attention to the moments of our days, is the fruit of our practice.

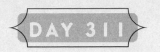

I rose this morning early as usual, and went to my desk. But it's spring, and the thrush is in the woods, somewhere in the twirled branches, and he is singing. And so now I am standing by the open door. And now I am stepping down onto the grass. I am touching a few leaves. I am noticing the way the yellow butterflies move together, in a twinkling cloud, over the field. And I am thinking: maybe just looking and listening is the real work. Maybe the world, without us, is the real poem.

Mary Oliver

To prepare myself to write this morning, I went for a short walk through my neighborhood to get a cup of coffee. I could have made coffee at home, but I wanted to stretch my legs and to breathe the fall air. As I walked, I allowed my neighborhood to entertain me with its colors, sounds, and smells. On my way back from the coffee shop, I saw a woman with a beautiful puppy, and I stopped to talk to her. She introduced herself as a student at my studio, and we discussed puppies as orange leaves drifted down around our heads. On my way home, I felt as if I was breathing in one of the last days of fall. *Dharana* is a decision we make to be present, to look and to listen, to allow ourselves to see and feel the words of the real poem.

I recently ran across a story about a Native American tribal leader describing his own inner struggles. He said, "There are two dogs inside me. One of the dogs is mean and evil. The other dog is good. The mean dog fights the good dog all the time." Someone asked him which dog usually wins, and after a moment's reflection, he answered, "The one I feed the most."

Rabbi Harold S. Kushner

I've found that the greatest motivator for consistent application of spiritual principles is pain. The memory of some recent failure, embarrassment, or anxiety supports me in my efforts to apply some forgotten truth to my life. To use the rabbi's example, it is only after feeding the evil dog that I am strongly persuaded to feed the good dog. Understanding this has taught me to appreciate the fiascos I've endured over the years as the learning experiences that they were. Because of my human capacity to learn from my mistakes, these experiences are the foundation on which my spiritual life has been built. The maintenance of my spiritual health reflects the stages of the eight-limb path. I think of *pratyahara* as the decision not to feed the evil dog. *Dharana* is the will to feed the good dog with consistency. There is a momentum in this process, which begins with pain but over time transforms into love. At first we're afraid of the evil dog, but over time we come to love the good dog. The power of this love for the good dog is the essence of *dharana*. This love we feel when we apply spiritual principles, when we share ourselves without reservation, is compelling. It sustains our attention, and sustained attention is *dharana*—and with sustained attention we can transform our world.

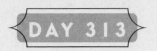
DAY 313

The real juice of life, whether it be sweet or bitter, is to be
found not nearly so much in the products of our efforts as in
the process of living itself, in how it feels to be alive.

George Leonard

Dharana is how it feels to be alive. Like a dog running across a field, we are
enthralled and fully engaged; all systems are go. This is my experience of
teaching yoga. There is a part of me that seems always to be afraid, another
part of me for which nothing seems ever to be enough—and yet there I
am, in a river of humanity, allowing myself to be seen and heard just as I
am, in the moment. Some days I move beyond this to *dhyana* and *samadhi,*
complete surrender of the self—but those moments are for another day. My
everyday experience of teaching is *dharana,* sustained attention, and it is
enough. It is entirely good to partake in life in this fashion, open to the
sweetness, open to the bitterness, open to giving, open to receiving, open
to how it feels to be alive.

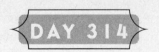
DAY 314

When you relinquish then you expand.

Zen master Dennis Genpo Merzel

In asana and meditation practice we have the opportunity to cultivate a sustained attention that we will be able to bring into our everyday lives. This is

all well and good, but first we have to develop that sustained attention on the mat or on the cushion. How is this accomplished? What do we have to do? The first step is always the same. We have to show up. We put the mat down, and we place our feet upon it. We set the timer, then sit our butts on the cushion. The second step is even simpler: we let go.

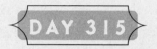

DAY 315

When the deepest currents of our life no longer have any influence on the waves at the surface, then our vitality will eventually ebb, and we will end up listless and bored even when we are busy.

Henri J. M. Nouwen

In the stillness of practice, we encounter the plane of existence where the one and the many are the same, where the limited self opens to the limitless. We move into what Henri J. M. Nouwen calls "the deepest currents of our lives." These currents are not of the physical plane, they are of spirit, encountered in moments of sustained attention, in deep states of concentration. Our minds and souls are immersed, connected, and we are at one with the universal mind, the universal spirit. We emerge from our practice forever changed by the experience. Our outlook is different; we have undergone the miracle of a shift in perspective. Regular practice generates a momentum as more of these experiences follow, one after the other. We feel our life force flowing ever more freely, wherever it is needed. The reverse is also true. Avoiding practice creates inertia. It is as if we each have a life muse, whose voice can be heard only in the stillness of practice, in the quiet of *dharana*. The inspiration with which we live our lives grows in relation to the frequency with which we visit our muse.

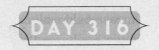

DHARANA

For what is prayer but the expansion of yourself into the living ether? . . . When you pray, you rise up to meet in the air those who are praying at that very hour, and whom save in prayer you may not meet. Therefore let your visit to that temple invisible be for naught but ecstasy and sweet communion.

Kahlil Gibran

Our practice is a visit to "that temple invisible." Over time, we train our minds to turn their focus inward, and to observe our inner world—the sensations of the body, the experience of breath, our mind's inner dialogue, the terrain of our emotional responses. Like a traveler discovering an uncharted land, we move into the invisible universe of our interior. The longer we are able to stay in this new land, the more powerfully we learn to concentrate, the more we find that our interior world is a shared one. Indeed, it is only the most external aspect of ourselves that is separate. As we draw inward, our intelligence comes in contact with Intelligence, our mind communes with Mind. This connection creates an energy, a vibration in our lives that accelerates our growth and is in fact the process whereby we become who we are meant to be.

Yogis in India stare at the sun (when it is first setting or rising only—it's not harmful to the eyes then). They hold the image of the sun in their mind's eye for practice of meditation. Once the form is established in the consciousness, the eyes are closed and the mental image of the flame or the holy figure is retained and transposed into our mind's eye.

Beryl Bender Birch

Yoga teacher Beryl Bender Birch gives us a crystal clear image of *dharana* when the object of concentration is internal. Just as we can use our own bodies as an external focus for *dharana,* so also can we bring our attention to an internal object, an image in the mind's eye, and use it to train the mind to concentrate deeply. The internal object I use most often when meditating is my heart. I bring my mind's eye to the center of my heart chakra, at the center of my chest, and hold my attention there, communing with the contents of my heart. Whether the focus is on an external or internal object is up to you; follow your own inclination on any given day. What is important to grasp is that, through regular practice, the mind's ability to concentrate grows, and this ability is the underpinning of all that we do in yoga.

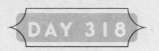

Concentration is sometimes identified with "one-pointedness" (*ekagrata*), but this is not quite correct, for the latter simply represents the arrest of the psycho mental flow, while concentration implies a fixation of the mind in order to gain understanding; as such, *dharana* is a creative act."

Georg Feuerstein

We apply our minds in the quiet of *dharana* to come to an understanding of what is. We have done this all our lives. Who has not squinted her eyes as she tried to catch a phone number spoken softly on an answering machine, or driven home on a dark, winding road, straining at the edge of her seat in an effort to see? Concentrating in order to gain insight is not a yogic invention. Nor is developing one's powers of concentration through physical training unique to yoga. The great sword masters of Japan, dancers, gymnasts, athletes of all kinds have developed their ability to concentrate while simultaneously developing their physical skills. Yoga has not introduced a new discipline, it has simply given us a new emphasis. In yoga practice, the mind's ability to concentrate is primary; the body's ability to master a posture is secondary. This is true because the nature of *dharana* is creative. As we apply our minds to the moment, a synergy happens between what is and what we have already experienced. An entirely new understanding becomes possible. New worlds open up. Evolution becomes possible.

DAY 319

*When I understood . . . I began to feel differently. The dark
void in my heart began to glimmer with the light of hope, and
the emptiness inside of me was replaced with the beginnings
of self-knowledge. I saw that the basic source of my discontent
was my mind, the attitudes I had chosen, and not what
other people had done to me.*

The Reverend Jesse Lee Peterson

What we find when we apply a concentrated mind to our world is that the truth has always been there, we have just been too distracted to know it. The world that opens up to us in our yoga practice has always been there. It is the world of Adam and Eve in the garden of Eden, the world of Jesus and the Buddha, the world of children and puppies. Our practice is a peeling back of the layers of delusion that stand between us and the true home of our spirit. The first step is cognitive. The addict wakes up one morning and *knows* that his drinking is the problem. Yesterday it was everything else, but on this morning he understands, in the deepest core of his soul, that all his problems start with a drink.

Most of our problems are more complex than this, but the solution always begins with a shift in perspective. The concentration we practice on the mat and on the meditation cushion taps us into the real information superhighway. We cannot spend time in *dharana* without accessing new insight. Sometimes it is insight about how to take out the trash, other times it is an idea for the screenplay you have been meaning to write, sometimes it is a deeper understanding of your place in the world. These insights, this inspiration, are an energy that has existed in the unmanifest realm and that comes into being through our thoughts, our words, and our deeds. Moving between two worlds, we become channels for grace in our own lives and the lives of others.

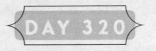

> Perhaps one of the greatest rewards of meditation and prayer is the sense of belonging that comes to us. We no longer live in a completely hostile world. We are no longer lost and frightened and purposeless. The moment we catch even a glimpse of God's will, the moment we begin to see truth, justice, and love as the real and eternal things in life, we are no longer deeply disturbed by all of the seeming evidence to the contrary that surrounds us.
>
> Bill Wilson

In *dharana,* mind connects to Mind, spirit connects to Spirit. Insight flows from this connection, but what keeps most of us returning to our mats and to our cushions is the peace that enters our lives as a result of becoming still.

Right below the surface of life is an ocean of spirit. *Dharana* penetrates everyday life and brings us into direct contact with this ocean. Whether we are sitting in meditation or working intently in a flower bed, the experience of sustained attention is peace. Bill Wilson describes the effects of this plainly and accurately. Freed from a self-imposed sense of separateness, we experience a visceral sense of belonging in a universe held together by love. Over time, this sense of being love in a universe of love becomes the rock upon which our spiritual lives are built. It gives us the ability to withstand the rigors of the life we were meant to live. It is the calmly abiding center from which all right action finds its source, and from it spring the acts of loving-kindness that will define our adult lives.

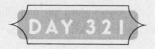
By nature Mercury and mind are unsteady: there is nothing in the world which cannot be accomplished when these are made steady.

Hatha Yoga Pradipika

In the early nineties I was trained as an addictions counselor. Brimming with the desire to help, I took a job with teenagers at a residential program. At the time, I knew nothing about teenagers, and nothing about residential programs either, for that matter. As it happens, residential programs for adolescents are about the hardest places to work on God's green earth. I should have guessed what I was in for when a young colleague told me with a straight face that he wanted a career in the Secret Service and had been told that this sort of work would put him in good stead.

Within six months, I was utterly wasted. I was awash with clinical responsibilities and I could not begin to understand how they were all going to be worked out. My most challenging task was a weekly substance-abuse group that I ran with a woman who could help out only occasionally. The students had never been in a group until I arrived on the scene, and they were by no means convinced that they had to show up for me. The creative challenges of the work were enormous; the emotional challenges were draining. As an escape from the near constant fear of failure I was living with, I began practicing yoga and meditation in earnest. As the months went by, I found that my ideas for the group had started to come more easily. Before I knew it, a vision had begun to form in my mind of the larger picture, as well as inspiration for the week-in, week-out format. As this vision energized me, I began to inspire some confidence in the students. Eventually, they were inspired by my vision as well. Over the course of four years, a cofacilitator and I created a comprehensive and effective program that we put into place in another center, as well as at the original one. I can't even guess at the number of young people directly affected by these programs, aspects of which are still in operation today, years after we've both moved on. I see these programs not as works of my own but as manifestations of grace moving through my practice and out into the world.

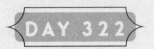

DAY 322

Have I walked long enough where the sea breaks raspingly
all day and all night upon the pale sand? Have I admired
sufficiently the little hurricane of the hummingbird?
The heavy thumb of the blackberry? The falling star?

Mary Oliver

There is a part of each of us that would like us to miss the point—a part of each of us that wants to believe that there will be no magic, no mystery, that our own life is not blessed and sacred, that our days are not a miracle, and that we are not connected to all living beings as a leaf is to a tree. In response to this predicament, we have created yoga.

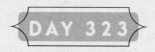

DAY 323

*I am the light of the world. Whoever follows me will never walk
in darkness but will have the light of life.*

John 8:12

We are all the light of the world. That is the point of spiritual practice—to reconnect to ourselves as the light of the world. *Dharana* is a dance we enter into with the real, with the light. First we choose to stop, then we bring all our mental powers of perception to one point. Our attention is a call that the universe responds to. In the stillness of a concentrated mind, a void is created where there had been mental chatter. The universe pours itself into that void, so that *dharana* is like a river that can flow in two directions. Our job is to create the void, to dig the well, to create emptiness so that the light of the world can pour in and through us.

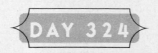

DAY 324

*The three grand essentials to happiness in life are something to
do, something to love, and something to hope for.*

Joseph Addison

Besides being a life-changing process, my yoga practice gives me a way to express my spirituality; it is my "something to do." By organizing my day around my practice, I place my spiritual well-being at the top of my to-do list. I accord my physical, mental, and spiritual health their rightful place in my life.

Teaching yoga, I discovered my "something to love." To be effective as a teacher, I must love everyone in the room. The moment I fail to do so, I block the flow of spirit in the class and become an impediment to the process of the class's unfolding. This requirement—to love each of the two-hundred-plus souls who come into my studio each day—offers me a profound opportunity for growth.

Teaching yoga has completed my journey. My students affirm daily all that is right about humanity. In so doing, they have given me "something to hope for." As I watch the everydayness, the commonplaceness, of their courage, their undeniable ability to surmount obstacles, I feel as though I am being given a glimpse of the answer. It is as if I have inside information about how all the big problems are going to be resolved. Who is going to address the environment, war, oppression, hopelessness? We are.

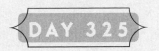

DAY 325

These three together—*dharana, dhyana,* and *samadhi*— constitute integration or *samyama.*

Yoga Sutras

Dharana, dhyana, and *samadhi* are viewed as a continuous flow of mind returning to Mind, spirit returning to Spirit. This movement, this flow to the glow, is called *samyama.* In the final sections, we will look at each aspect, each state of consciousness, individually because they are discrete occurrences, each with its own properties and its own contribution to our spiritual health, but I will also refer to them collectively as *samyama,* because they are in fact one movement.

In yogic philosophy, our souls first manifest as mineral or rock, then evolve into vegetation, then into animals, and finally assume human form. As this evolution occurs there is an acceleration, the process speeds up, light returning to Light. As humans we undertake spiritual practice in order to finish the journey home. In yoga there is a final, timeless moment in this process, one that has spanned countless lifetimes, and that is what we know as *samyama.*

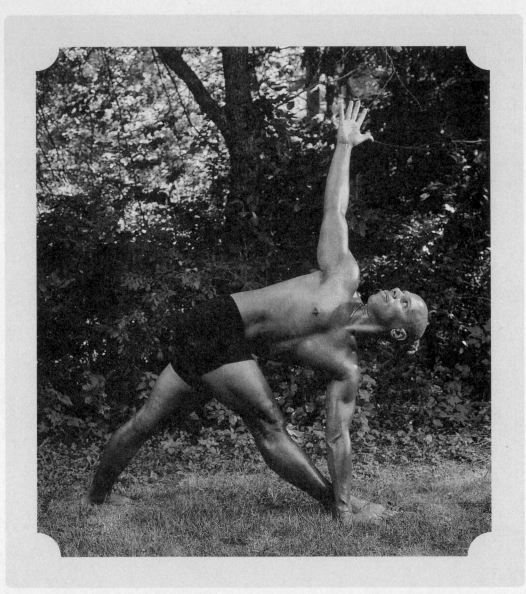

PART SEVEN

DHYANA

Effortless Attention

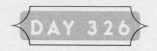
DAY 326

A steady continuous flow of attention directed towards
the same point or region is meditation.

Yoga Sutras

The seventh aspect of yoga's eight-limb path is meditation, or *dhyana*. Once we have learned to practice *dharana,* to quiet the mind through focused effort, something else begins to happen. We can already bring our mind to one point and keep it there; we have an awareness of the mind and the object of concentration, the seer and the seen. Now, *dharana* leads to *dhyana,* attention becomes effortless, there is no longer a seer, only the seen. We experience this kind of effortless absorption in love when our love for our child or partner transcends all thoughts of our personal safety or comfort. Because it is an intrinsic aspect of our nature, we also experience *dhyana* in our everyday activities. As a waiter, I would count the tables I was assigned at the beginning of the evening. "I have two tables," then, "I have four tables." After long months of practice, I came to understand that I was not truly working until I no longer knew or cared how many tables I had. At that point, I was simply in flow. There was only the moment, and the next right task to perform. Counting tables was *dharana,* and *dharana* became *dhyana* when the tables disappeared and there was only the task.

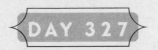

In *dhyana*, psychological and chronological time come to a standstill as the mind observes its own behavior. The intensity of attention in the field of consciousness neither alters nor wavers, remaining as stable, smooth, and constant as oil pouring from a jug. Maintaining the same intensity of awareness, the attentive awareness moves from one-pointed concentration to no pointed attentiveness . . . in *dhyana* the emphasis is on the maintenance of a steady and profound contemplative observation.

B. K. S. Iyengar

It is important to understand that *dharana* and *dhyana* are skills we can cultivate. In fact, the eight-limb path itself and the names given these states of mind were established long after the fact. The Yoga Sutras are simply describing experiences that human beings had already been having for centuries. The point of understanding the difference between *dharana* and *dhyana* is that our understanding can inform the way we approach any endeavor. Think of *dharana* and *dhyana* as aspects of the anatomy of excellence in action. Equipped with a model of how we and others have achieved excellence, we can better prepare ourselves to live our dreams. *Dhyana* is that profound place that sports psychologists call "the zone." It is that place where the musician and her instrument disappear and there is only the music; the timeless place in which the public speaker no longer speaks from knowledge but from an unerring sense of the moment. Through fearlessness and dedication we leave behind the everyday impediments and enter the realm of pure energy, pure spirit, unerring right action. All of us have the capacity to live from this place if we practice.

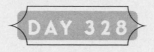

He should lift up the self by the Self.

Bhagavad Gita

We embark on a remarkable journey as we begin to consciously flow through the stages of *samyama*—from concentration to meditation, from meditation to *samadhi*. This is a journey powered by spirit. We do not attempt to make *dhyana* a regular part of our experience for selfish reasons, or with the will of the unaided ego. Rather, we prepare ourselves to be open to grace. With the *yamas* and the *niyamas* serving as the rock upon which all our efforts rest, we become willing to be used by love for love's purposes. So motivated, we cannot fail. Our hearts and minds untroubled, we are able to apply ourselves in the service of others unstintingly. This unswerving dedication flows from *dharana* to *dhyana*. We find that our practice and our lives are imbued with divine energy. Whatever work or relationships may come our way, they are transformed by the grace that flows through us. Our own experience of being in the world is one of ever-increasing peace, clarity, understanding, and ability. We are no longer acting solely on our own behalf; rather, we have become channels for grace.

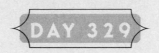

Use your own light, and return to the source of light,
that is called practicing eternity.

Lao-Tzu

Halfway around the world, in another time and place, a different sage has come to the same conclusion as Krishna in the Bhagavad Gita. We turn our attention inward to discover our own light, and our own light guides us to the source of light. We take one step toward the light, and the light takes ten steps toward us. As a military parachutist, I spent weeks learning how to properly exit an airplane—only to find that once I was near enough to the exit, I would be unceremoniously sucked out by the 180-miles-per-hour wind howling by the door. Much of the time we spend mastering technique is similar to the time I spent learning how to properly exit an aircraft. Once we do become still, the power of stillness draws us inward. Our own light guides us to the source of light.

The mind generally takes up various objects, runs into all sorts
of things. That is the lower state. There is a higher state of the
mind, when it takes up one object and excludes all others.

Swami Vivekananda

In yogic scriptures, the same point is made over and over again. The distracted mind has no power, the directed mind has limitless potential. Most
of the work we do in yoga precedes *dhyana*. It may take years, and seemingly endless diligence, before you can curb your restless mind and bring it
to bear on the things that make life worthwhile. But the time you'll spend
in *dhyana,* with a directed mind, will increase as you practice.

Each of us finds his or her own most effective technique for taming the
mind. You may find that meditation works for you; others achieve stillness
and concentration in asana practice or *pranayama*. I find it by teaching asana.
The requirements of teaching yoga have proved a very effective device for
bringing my mind to one point and keeping it there. For me, the point of
meditation in teaching is my intuition. Just as we follow the breath in meditation, or observe bodily sensation in asana, when I teach, I watch the
impulses of intuition and inspiration as they arise. I observe the nature of
each impulse and its relationship to the moment: "This one is inspired by
the group energy." "This one is inspired by a momentary pause in the flow
of my attention and it should not be heeded, but rather be taken as a sign
that I need to bring my mind back." "This one is a pure empathic hit of
what their bodies would like right now." And so on. While I'm teaching,
my attention is steady and continuous, and concentration is by and large
effortless—there is no past, no future, only a timeless present. I am in *dhyana*.
Having come into *dhyana* over and over again in this fashion, I can carry the

experience over into other areas of my life. In writing, asana practice, public speaking, and other forms of teaching, I now have the ability to drop into *dhyana* because it has become a place my mind moves to with ease. The effects of practice are progressive and cumulative. Health radiates out from that center like rings rippling out across the surface of a lake.

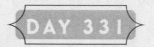

DAY 331

Only if you are able to be conscious without thought can you use your mind creatively, and the easiest way to enter that state is through your body. Whenever an answer, a solution, or a creative idea is needed, stop thinking for a moment by focusing attention on your inner energy field. Become aware of the stillness. When you resume thinking, it will be fresh and creative. In any thought activity, make it a habit to go back and forth every few minutes or so between thinking and an inner kind of listening, an inner stillness. We could say: don't just think with your head, think with your whole body.

Eckhart Tolle

As my teaching has progressed, I have learned to think with my whole body. I've increasingly expanded my awareness to include the information coming to me from the rest of my body. My emotional reactions and my physical sensations play an integral part in the ongoing assessment I'm making as I guide a class. Through the power of repetition and unwavering attention, I have come to know an ever-increasing number of paths to understanding. I go down the wrong path and I am blocked. I do this again, but this time my attention registers the faint impulse that has led me here before, and this impulse now becomes a road sign. As we grow in self-awareness, we grow in effectiveness. The clarity and stillness of *dhyana* compresses time and speeds our development, but our growth still depends on our willingness to let go, to have faith. I can think with my whole body, but without faith I will not act on what I know. Insight must be matched with faith.

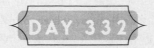

Though my view is as spacious as the sky, my actions and respect
for cause and effect are as fine as grains of flour.

Padmasambhava

In *samyama* our practice is bearing fruit that can be fully realized only in action. We have created spaciousness in our bodies, our minds, and our hearts so that divinity can flow into that space and out into the world, through our thoughts, on our lips, and with our hands.

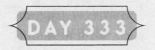

Architects of social policy who have stayed in air-conditioned
offices have rarely created programs that are well tuned to the
needs of the poor or others who need their help.

Mirabai Bush

Deep states of concentration, long periods of restful, meditative reflection, or ecstatic periods of oneness have no enduring value without love. Each one of us is called to put love into action. It is up to you, up to me, up to all of us to be the teacher who cared, the hand that reached out, the voice that said no or yes, the Samaritan who pulled over and offered assistance on the side of the road. I read recently of a paramedic who woke up on September 11, 2001, to the news that the World Trade Center had been hit by aircraft. He went down to the site of the tragedy and, after tunneling for twelve hours deep in the rubble, saved the last person who was taken alive from the wreckage. He did not think of himself as extraordinary, and so it was two months before this story even made it into the newspapers. This is the grace that only we, ordinary men and women, can bring into the world. And it is for this that we spend time on our mats and our cushions.

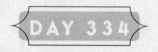

DAY 334

How can we live in the present moment, live right now with the people around us, helping to lesson their suffering and making their lives happier? How? The answer is we must practice mindfulness.

Thich Nhat Hanh

The spacious, steady attention of *dhyana* is meant to be the foundation upon which we can build more effective lives. Watching the truly proficient—the great comedians, teachers, actors, leaders, artisans, and athletes—we get the sense that they have ascended to a place of unerring understanding. There is no uncertainty; their minds have been absorbed by Mind, their spirits rest in Spirit.

When I'm at my best as a teacher, there is always a moment—sometimes as I am walking through the door into the room, other times shortly after we begin—when the class comes to me as a fully formed idea. I could not tell you what the idea is or what posture we are going to do when; I know only that the message has been received. There is nothing more for me to do. It is as though I have traveled through time and seen how this particular class turns out. I get a glimpse of how time is not linear, of how everything is happening all at once in the mind of God; the beginning, the middle, and the end has already happened and is happening now. Our practice attunes us to the knowing we need in order to be the people we want to be.

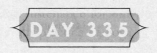

DAY 335

What would you do if you weren't afraid?

Spencer Johnson, M.D.

In some ways this is a trick question, because when you are in *dhyana* you are not afraid. But it is a helpful question, too, because most of us are often not in *dhyana,* and confronting our fear helps to broaden our perspective. As you consider your own answer to this question, you can see once again the power of training the mind in asana, *pranayama,* and meditation. Time spent on our mats or on our meditation cushions has the potential to be time spent when we are not afraid. From the vantage point of our practice, we are able to view our lives without the corrosive influence of fear. As the mind becomes accustomed to stillness, we are able to move out of fear and into stillness with increasing skill and ease. The fear that is a product of our distracted mind loses its significance and becomes no more than an indication that we have not been paying attention. Fear is our reminder to resume living in the real. We begin to know what we would do if we were not afraid.

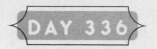

Every meditation technique has one object as its focal point that you return to again and again. It could be the breath, a mantra, a thought, a sensation, a prayer. Having sensation in the body as the focal point is a powerful doorway for the mind to be drawn inside. The first level is concentration, or *dharana*. I see this as being one-pointed, and it is very much associated with the linear mind. We naturally move into altered states, and sometimes we will experience *dhyana*, or what could be called "one-flowingness," and in this flowingness we become more aware of the field in which the thoughts are arising.

Sudhir Jonathan Foust

Tracing our thoughts back to their origin is a profound practice. Actively cultivating the ability to do this in the moment has limitless potential for our spiritual health. In so doing, we become adults. Without this skill, we are grown-up children, prey to each passing desire and aversion, every fear and ambition. By teaching our minds spaciousness and concentration, and then turning our attention inward, so that our moment-to-moment internal reality can be perceived and understood, we extricate ourselves from our past conditioning.

Two scenarios: In one, you are talking to someone who both frightens and angers you. You spend the conversation managing these feelings, and you make your exit as soon as possible. In the second scene, you've had a shift in perspective. You are connected to your own light and you have faith in who you are. Nevertheless, you have the same negative reaction to this person. But in this second scenario, you abide calmly and see clearly. You observe your reaction to this person and trace it to its origin. You understand that neither you nor this person need be accountable to your old beliefs about yourself and others. In the spaciousness of this attitude, you allow yourself to be present and to be open to this person as a child of God. In other words, in the second scenario, you are able to behave like an adult. Growth on the mat is growth.

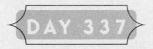

DAY 337

It is very important, especially while you are young, to love something with your whole being—a tree, an animal, your teacher, your parent—for then you will find out for yourself what it is to be without conflict, without fear.

J. Krishnamurti

We are moving into a fearless place, the foundation of which is love. Without love, technique becomes an empty exercise devoid of spiritual content or energetic potency. All the adjectives used to describe *dhyana* are attributes of love. The steady, unbroken flow of attention is animated by love— love of oneself, love for one's place in the universe, love for all beings. Without love we will fatigue, lose interest, lose heart. Before I met my wife, I was the same person that I am today. I had the same abilities, the same smile, many of the same hopes and dreams. But I had not lived up to my potential, and by and large I didn't care. It wasn't that I quit anything; I just hadn't really tried anything that would require me to truly grow. Over the last seven years, my wife and I have grown steadily, moving from one blistering challenge to the next. We often laugh at the sheer difficulty of some of the situations that we have said yes to during the time we've been together; the trials have been nonstop. But the universe knows we are ready, because we have each other. In the context of our love for each other, all our efforts, all the days we walk out into the unknown make sense. The clarity, spaciousness, connectedness, power, insight, and compassion that we are awakening in our practice is love.

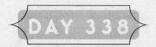

With the loss of time comes the complete absence of ordinary identity. The personality that I feel myself to be dissolves beyond the material level, and with that, I lose the need for the landmarks that I have gathered since birth.

Deepak Chopra

The phrase "When I grow up" is a powerful indicator that we are born with a sense of spiritual potential. I believe we each possess an intuitive understanding that our limited self, created in fear and defined by suffering, is not our destiny. Rather, there is a grown-up self waiting for us just around the corner. The corner is turned by a combination of insight and action. Many people gain insight without actually seeking it; the apostle Paul, on the road to Damascus, is one of the best-known examples. But even Paul's dramatic encounter would have been for naught had he not followed it up with courageous action. The aim of spiritual practice is to deliberately cultivate insight and to instill in ourselves the strength we need for courageous action. *Dhyana* is a place where action and insight become one. When we are in this state of sustained focus and flow, the action of attention and the insight gained from detached observation occur simultaneously. Here, in this timeless still point, we grow up. In the presence of the real, of truth, we are no longer interested in our constructed personalities. The fears and desires of our fabricated self are forgotten, as is the small talk we were engaged in moments before hearing the news of a birth or a death. *Dhyana* is both. We find that in the timeless realm of the spirit, we were always grown up.

> DAY 339

> The *samskaras* are built up by continued action of the thought-waves, and they, in their turn, create new thought-waves, the process works both ways. Expose the mind to constant thoughts of anger and resentment, and you will find that these anger-waves build-up anger-samskaras, which will predispose you to find occasions for anger throughout your daily life. A man with well developed anger-samskaras is said to have "a bad temper." The sum total of our samskaras is, in fact, our character at any given moment.
>
> Yoga Sutras

In yogic psychology, our predispositions, the contents of our character, are in a state of perpetual cocreation with our thoughts. Our thoughts create impressions on our souls, *samskaras,* and these impressions, in turn, predispose us to similar thoughts. Over time, these impressions can become quite pronounced, as in the case of addiction. But like impressions made on the surface of a candle, our *samskaras* can be melted away by heat. The heat we apply is yoga. *Dharana* and *dhyana,* whether experienced in asana, *pranayama,* meditation, or some other activity, are so powerful because they bring us to a place beyond thought and the impressions of thought, and into *vidya,* direct knowledge of the soul. Our thoughts can refashion our *samskaras;*

dharana and *dhyana* eliminate our preconceived notions altogether. As Deepak Chopra so eloquently articulated in the last essay, we can move beyond our self-created personalities, let go of our self-limiting definitions, and realize our true nature.

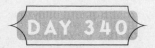

DAY 340

> Writing of Bernard Goetz, the man who shot four teenage boys on a New York subway in 1984, Lillian Rubin claimed that his bullets were "aimed at targets that existed as much in his past as in his present."
>
> Malcolm Gladwell

We live in a shadow world, where the past flits about the present, glimpsed out of the corner of our eyes, just beyond reach. Our boss is a composite of our mother and father and the peer group we both loved and hated. The thing we fear the most is the thing we most need. We make statements that are questions and ask questions that are statements, reveal ourselves to strangers and hide ourselves from the people we love. Bernard Goetz is said to have sought out an environment that confirmed his worst fears, and then to have desperately tried to redress the wrongs of his imagined world. How different are we from him? And how does yoga change this?

Yoga works from the outside in. We begin with a study of our actions, move on to our bodies, and on to our breath. Then, turning inward, we follow our thoughts to their source. We use our own light to return to the source of light. With our attention resting steadily in the present, our bondage to past conditioning slowly dissipates. Who we thought we were slowly fades into unimportance in the brilliant light of our true nature.

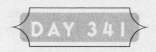

When asked whether he was a god or a man,
Buddha replied, simply, "I am awake."

Lama Surya Das

I spend a good portion of my days worried about some outcome: "How will that turn out?" "What if I don't measure up?" This often leads to some form of anger. "Why can't that person just drive?" "Mariam, where did you put the phone? Why can't you put the phone back where it belongs?" The anger often leads to depression: "I am just going to spend the rest of my life being an asshole." Then I see my dog lying on our couch. She looks up at me, smiles, and wags her tail. I hug her, smelling her warm fur, feeling how good it is to love something, to give love and to receive love. I experience reality. I am awake.

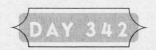

The Japanese word *zen, ch'an* in Chinese, *dhyana* in Sanskrit,
means meditation. Zen aims, through meditation, to realize
what Buddha himself realized, the emancipation of one's mind.

Paul Reps and Nyogen Senzaki

In the contemplative traditions, the emancipation of one's mind is gained through stillness and connection. In yoga, the body and the breath are used to accomplish this. Motionless in a posture, breathing into our physical, emotional, and psychic experience of the moment, we are profoundly present, still, and connected. I go through periods when I minimize the contemplative aspects of asana, only to return with wonder at the realization of just how profoundly anchoring my asana practice is. In my studio, which is my business, surrounded by students, who are also my customers, in the middle of a day that started at 6:30 A.M. and won't be over until 10 P.M., I pause. I am in awe at how at ease I am, at home in my body, my mind absorbed by the details of my practice. *Pratyahara, dharana, dhyana,* steady, effortless, flowing attention. I am free to be where I am, doing what I am doing, with a mind that is clear and untroubled and a heart that is at ease.

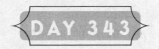

DAY 343

Concentrate your mind on me, fill your heart with my presence.

Bhagavad Gita

Earlier I said that the internal point of focus I use most often in meditation is my heart. This is true, but the one I love the most is God. My favorite meditation is to simply sit with my heart and my mind open to God's love. "Freight trains of love" is the phrase I use. Opening my heart and my mind to freight trains of love, I sit still and let the light pour into my soul. This is worthwhile.

DAY 344

You live in illusion and the appearance of things. There is a reality, but you do not know this. When you understand this, you will see that you are nothing. And being nothing, you are everything. That is all.

Kalu Rinpoche

Being nothing isn't all that bad. It means we are one with everything. There is no separation between you and a beautiful lake or meadow. You are summer clouds, beautiful and free. You stalk jungle trails with the strength and silence of a jaguar, and you float along on currents of air like a hawk. There is no unrequited love, no loss, for all beings are a family; we have always been together and we will always be together. We cannot fail. And we are never alone.

When I began teaching big classes, I knew that I was not a good enough teacher. I looked at all those people, crowded together in a hot room, and I felt how badly they wanted a great class. But it was impossible for me to give it to them; I just would not be able to pull it off. Then, one day, I realized that I didn't have to.

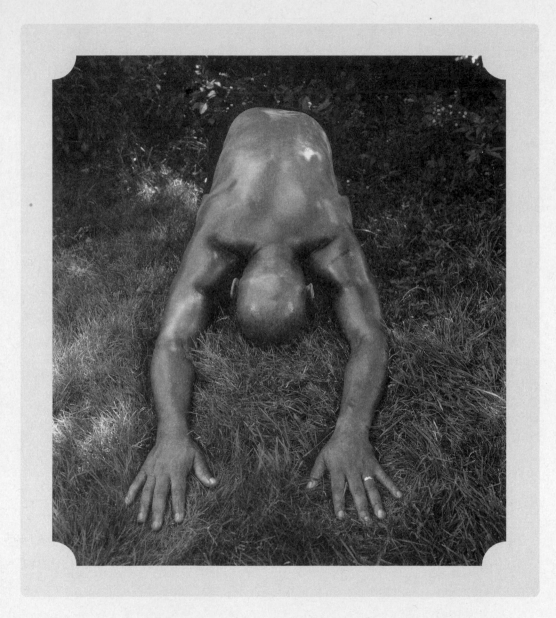

PART EIGHT

SAMADHI

Self-Forgetting

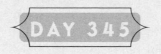

Who are we, not to shine?

Nelson Mandela

The final aspect of the yoga path is *isvara-pranidhana,* or surrender to God. Faith, surrender, devotion. Faith in what? Surrender to what? Devotion to what? The answers to these questions cannot be found in any book, they are written in our hearts. They were written long before we were born, and we practice yoga to complete our journey back to the truth about our-selves. Whether or not you have a God or want a God is irrelevant. All of us have experienced moments of profound connectedness—the caress of a spring breeze on bare skin, the feeling in our chests when we look into another's eyes with love, the holy awe of gazing at a star-strewn summer sky. There is a greatness right beneath the surface of everyday life, and every once in a while we catch a glimpse of it. Those are the sudden, lucid flashes when life beguiles us out of the prison of our minds and leads us right into the moment. On our mats and on our meditation cushions, we begin to expe-rience this deep connectedness as an everyday occurrence. *Isvara-pranidhana* is about making the experience of that greatness a priority.

And why not? We can live in the light with the same ease with which we live in our darkness. We are surrounded by mentors, by men and women who have chosen to live life on a higher plane, for a higher purpose. The music we listen to, the movies we watch, the books we read—all abound with references to the sweetness of "amazing grace." This final moment in the eight limbs of yoga is about allowing grace to happen. Not hoping for it to happen, not trying hard to let it happen, not believing that one day it will happen—this final moment is about letting it happen. It is about shin-ing, and who are we not to shine?

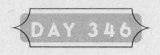

All that is necessary to make this world a better place to live is to love, to love as Christ loved, as Buddha loved.

Isadora Duncan

Samadhi, the eighth and final limb, is the experience of ecstatic oneness. In and of itself it is, for most of us, simply a pleasant reality, like a good blueberry muffin. The lesson of *samadhi,* however, is that it can be reached only through self-forgetting, and that lesson can be applied in all things. As I write these words, my life is taken up with finishing this book, directing a large urban yoga studio, preparing to open an even larger studio in Boston, and looking for a new place to live. I feel inadequate to all of these tasks, but I also know that God isn't interested in my opinion of her works. I will continue to serve in my own inadequate fashion until God fires me, because what God is doing is more important than my neurotic fears and discomfort. And I find that as the Prayer of Saint Francis says, "Through self-forgetting we find." Through self-forgetting I can love as Christ did, I can love as Buddha did.

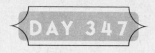

> When the object of meditation engulfs the meditator, appearing as the subject, self-awareness is lost. This is *samadhi.*
>
> Yoga Sutras

In attempting to tease out the moment when *dhyana* becomes *samadhi,* we understand why the ancients grouped *dharana, dhyana,* and *samadhi* under the word *samyama.* The musician who has lost herself in her music passes from *dharana* to *dhyana,* glimpses *samadhi* in ecstatic moments, and returns to *dharana*—all in the space of a song. Each moment is an authentic realization of an aspect of *samyama.* The tenuousness of all of this is in our attachment to the ego. As the one who is playing the music, we really are not up to sustained *samadhi.* It is only after we have let go of our self-created identity and become nothing that we can remain in *samadhi.*

Though this might seem like unattainable spiritual acrobatics, in fact we have all experienced intentional ego deaths for a good cause. The most common is the adult's sacrifice of ego identification on behalf of children under her care. Teachers and parents are effective only to the extent that they can let go of outworn self-definitions, allowing themselves to be used by life, to be defined by the needs of the moment. The self-sacrifice of police officers and firefighters is another example of our human ability to subjugate our ego's survival to the needs of a good cause.

As yogis, we have defined spiritual growth as a good cause. Our commitment to our own spiritual health is so profound that we are willing to endure the many fears we experience on the way to becoming nothing. And that is what blocks us. We are afraid of being nothing, of letting go of who we have thought we are. To remain in *samadhi,* the state of oneness, we must die to the condition of separateness. The final step in the transformational process called yoga is possible only when we have let go of being who we think we are.

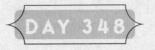

DAY 348

We don't know the reasons that propel us on a spiritual
journey, but somehow our life compels us to go. Something
in us knows that we are not just here to toil at our work.
There is a mysterious pull to remember.

Jack Kornfield

As children we sacrificed for our pets, for the sports we loved, for our hobbies, for success in school. As adults we have spent many a cold, dark night without sleep or food or acknowledgment, giving our all to some project because we thought it was the right thing to do. It is our human nature to endure hardship for a higher vision, a greater good. Eventually this aspect of our character becomes focused inward. Instead of sacrificing to see that the world has something better, we work to see that we have something better. The results we are seeking are not material; they are emotional, psychic, spiritual. We work to become at ease in our own skin, to become more loving, to understand. Those of us who have spent time at this discover a couple of paradoxes. The first is that our new thing is the oldest thing. Our many loves have been with the one love, the love beneath all loves. We are not trying something new when we become spiritual, we are remembering who we have always been. The second paradox we come to understand is that business as usual will not work. To better ourselves, we must stop thinking of ourselves. We cannot continue to be at the center of our lives. As children, we knew that love meant walking our dog even when we did not want to; as adults, we learn that we must be love even when we do not want to. We come to know that we are like the river, finding its fulfillment by vanishing into the ocean.

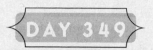

Because she has let go, she can care for the people's welfare as a mother cares for her child.

Lao-Tzu

For inspiration this morning, I've been listening to Tracy Chapman's first album, released in 1988. Much of the suffering she was singing about then still exists today, but I realize that many things have changed for the better as well. Our culture simply does not have the tolerance for the physical abuse of women that it had then. Help is more accessible for women; there are more effective programs for men who have been violent; as a society we have become more informed. It did not hurt that an outstanding artist, in her smash-hit debut album, addressed this issue in several of her songs.

In her own way Tracy Chapman succeeded in alleviating some of the pain of those around her. She simply practiced her art and dedicated it to the service of others. She had no idea what kind of impact her work would have. But she did it anyway, and she put it out there with all her heart and soul. By doing so, she made it that much easier for the rest of us to do the same.

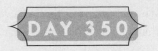

You stand in awe of what God has wrought, and in doing so,
you are worshipping Him who made you and inviting Him
to continue to remold your life and maintain control over
your destiny. The windows of heaven will open and you
will experience such an outpouring of abundance and
blessing that you will hardly have room to receive it.

Roy Masters

The essence of *samadhi* is profound connection. We "stand in awe of what God has wrought." Standing in awe is not only paying attention, it is entering into dialogue with creation. We are letting down the barriers to communication. The beauty that we see fills us, and we in turn can pour that beauty back out into the world. I have seen lakes in Maine that only a few human beings on earth have seen, but you do not need to go to them to feel their essence. Those lakes are in my heart, and by being with me, you can be with them. This is who we are to one another. And this is what the world is to us. We need only open our hearts and make room to receive it.

DAY 351

> Free from the "I" and "mine," from aggression, arrogance,
> greed, desire, and anger, he is fit for the state of absolute
> freedom. Serene in this state of freedom, beyond all
> desire and sorrow, seeing all beings as equal.
>
> Bhagavad Gita

Is this possible? I think so. I have come to believe that "I" and "mine," aggression, arrogance, greed, desire, and anger are mistakes that we can stop making. As the Bhagavad Gita suggests, a more perfect understanding of who we are will place us beyond the concepts of desire and sorrow, and once we know who we are, we can see all beings as equal. Until then, though, there will be pain, because we are not operating with all the facts at our disposal. We look out into the world and become confused. With one foot in delusion and the other in grace, we experience conflict, sadness, and the constraints of time.

Some of us, however, have moved beyond delusion, let go of our false personas, and spent time in direct contact with the underlying reality. Some people have called that experience *samadhi*. Those moments of connection and deep understanding support the notion of spiritual growth, spiritual health. Our situation is dynamic, we are ever changing, and if we listen to the promptings of our hearts and act with faith, we will grow up and become adults, in the true sense of the word.

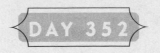

For as he thinketh in his heart, so is he.

Proverbs 23:7

My body had hardened around an image I had of myself. This image wasn't fully formed and it wasn't fully conscious, but it was constant, so my body conformed to it. I was stiff here, weak there, strong here, broken in other places—all according to the character I had made up for myself. In order to move through a series of asana that required my body to perform a normal range of motions, I had to confront the ways in which I had shut down to certain movements and eliminated certain options, in an attempt to maintain my self-made identity. Over the years, as I've melted away the stiffness, strengthened the weakness, and mended the broken places, I've also had to confront the mental, emotional, and spiritual assumptions that had created disability in my body where there could have been ability. In a parallel process, my mind and psyche have freed themselves of their own rigidity, weakness, and injuries. Gradually, over time, I've become capable of tolerating deeper and deeper levels of stillness and connection. As my body, mind, and spirit were gradually being redefined, what I thought in my heart changed as well, and so I changed.

SAMADHI

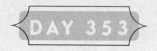

Ultimately, care of the soul results in an individual "I"
I never would have planned for or maybe even wanted.
By caring for the soul faithfully, every day, we step
out of the way and let our full genius emerge.

Thomas Moore

The theme of this final section is stepping out of the way, letting it happen. Thomas Moore reminds us that our souls need nurturing; they require faithful, day-in, day-out care. In yoga, we call this practice. Our practice makes it possible for us to get out of our own way. To a remarkable extent, I have actually been able to get out of my own way over the last few years, as I have grown into my adulthood.

I have gone from apprentice to journeyman in many areas of my life, and with this transition has come resistance. A part of me has become very comfortable in the apprentice role, and I have unconsciously resisted any changes that threaten my place in the world. This resistance has manifested itself in innumerable promptings from my ego to take drastic action: "By God, I am going to give her a piece of my mind." "This situation is intolerable! I am out of here!" "They won't have me to kick around anymore." You get the idea. My fear attempts to walk the world disguised as anger.

In the midst of my practice, though, the urge to do is replaced by the urge to wait and see. Suddenly, anger no longer feels like a wise or appropriate response. In the light of my practice, I decide that I would rather see how things turn out without my contribution. This simple shift in attitude has helped me avoid innumerable mistakes and fiascos that would have surely landed me back in the apprentice role again. With regular practice, regular care, I have been able to move forward in my life. The genius that is in my soul has risen closer to the surface.

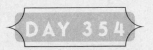

One beautiful June afternoon, as I stood on my ladder, I was overcome with a feeling of what I can only describe as profound and utter well-being. For no apparent reason, I dropped through some unexpected crack in my ordinary mode of consciousness into a state of "time out of time." The most mundane moments were infused with the deepest sense of satisfaction. The enchanting perfume of the iris at my feet; the steady hum of farm machinery in the distant field; the cat curled up in the sun, watching; even the rich oil smell of the paint. It all seemed so completely right. I was utterly OK.

Stephen Cope

Ecstatic oneness. Stephen Cope's description of his experience of entering *samadhi* while painting a house one summer is so compelling because the images he describes are at once so ordinary and yet so haunting in their crystalline clarity. He is recounting an experience we have all had, and yet have probably discounted and relegated to our subconscious. Reading this deeply evocative passage, we can't help but pause and reevaluate our own experiences, our own sacred moments of knowing that we are utterly OK, that all is right with the world—the afternoon in the forest, the dawn on a river, the timeless morning spent absorbed with a task. I actually had a similar experience painting a friend's kitchen over Christmas break one year. I have never had much aptitude for painting before or since, but the deep *samyama* I experienced during those winter days facilitated a patient competence that I marvel at to this day. We have all known such moments. The question is, what do we learn from them?

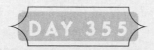

Liberation comes when the Yogi has fulfilled the *purusarthas,*
the fourfold aims of life.

Yoga Sutras

Near the beginning of this book I talked about the *purusarthas,* the four aims of life. Let us now use them as a means by which to evaluate the place *samadhi* has in our lives. The four aims are *dharma,* or duty; *artha,* or worldly purpose; *kama,* or enjoyment; and *moksa,* or liberation. *Dharma,* in this sense, is the duty that we have to ourselves. To use Thomas Moore's words again, it is the "care" we must take of our souls. How does yoga in general, and *samadhi* in particular, aid us in care of the soul?

The simplest answer lies in another question: "When does it not?" I believe we can hide out in yoga. We can use our practice as a way to hide from the necessary pain of life. We can also justify selfish acts with fanciful yogic notions: "He does not respect my practice, therefore I do not have to treat him with compassion or with respect." That said, if we show up on our mats and in our lives with integrity and good intentions, there is no aspect of our yoga practice that does not promote the care of our souls. All of the limbs of yoga either support that which is pleasing to the soul or bring us into direct knowledge of the soul, as in *samadhi.* If we are actively practicing the eight limbs of yoga, we are performing our duty to ourselves and living our *dharma.* It is that simple.

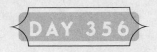

When he was a young man imprisoned in Cell 54, a solitary cell
in Cairo Central Prison . . . [Anwar Sadat] learned to withdraw
from his own mind and look at it, to see if the scripts were
appropriate and wise. He learned how to vacate his own mind
and, through a deep personal process of meditation, to work
with his own scriptures, his own form of prayer, and re-script
himself. . . . When he became president of Egypt and
confronted the political realities of his time, he re-scripted
himself towards Israel. He visited the Knesset in Jerusalem
and opened up one of the most precedent-breaking peace
movements in history. . . . Sadat was able to use his self-
awareness, his imagination and his conscience, to exercise
personal leadership, to change an essential paradigm,
to change the way he saw a situation.

Stephen R. Covey

The second aim in life is *artha,* or worldly purpose, meaning the role we
choose to play in our own lives and the lives of others. Anwar Sadat's experience of *samyama* changed his life and uplifted humanity. The work we do
can change water into wine when it is infused with the love we find at the
center of our being. We do not fulfill the aim of *artha* by having a job, writing a check, or participating in local politics. We fulfill the aim of *artha*
when the work that we do, the way we relate to the people in our lives, the
decisions that we make at every level reflect our deepest beliefs. *Dharma* is
the work we do to connect to our true selves; *artha* is sharing our true selves
with all beings.

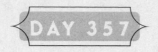

> I taught a class last night, and the students came in all scattered
> and going every which way. And you know, at the end of class,
> they were all close to the bone, and they had eyes that were
> bright and clear. That hour and forty minutes, it was miraculous.
> It was a kind of joint feeling in the room. Sixty people came in
> with all their different stories, and afterward they were all
> saying they were amazed, amazed by their own tranquillity.
> There is something about being close to the bone.
>
> Eleanor W., yoga teacher

I think that *kama,* the enjoyment of life, is at the heart of why yoga has become so popular in the United States. Yoga teaches us how to enjoy life, how to work, and how to rest. Most of the forces in our lives telling us how to work and how to play have a vested interest in the outcome. The airlines want us to fly, the travel agents want us to travel, our bosses want us to work for less than they are paid. Yoga is indifferent. It is like a tree in the middle of a vast forest—it just is, and it is nothing. The information we encounter in yoga is our own. Yoga does not enhance or diminish us, it simply reflects us back to ourselves as we are. One of the truths we discover in the mirror of yoga is that we are often unhappy, and that most of the time there is something we can do about it.

For me these days, *kama* has two great teachings. The first is not to take anything personally, least of all myself. The second is to let go. I come to the mat scattered, with many different stories about how I should take this personally or hold on to that. Then I spend time connecting to my body, to my breath, time "close to the bone." At the end of my practice I am amazed— I am experiencing joy, a joy that I am learning to bring out into the world.

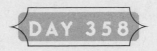
Before yoga, I worked out a lot. I was a workout maniac, the
harder the better. Then one day I woke up with sciatica pain
down my leg. I thought it would go away, but it got worse and
worse for the next two years. I couldn't work, sit down, or stand
up. I went to all the doctors and tried everything from deep
massage to chiropractors. Finally I quit the gym and went to
yoga. I lost weight, and after three months 75 percent of the
pain was gone. Then came other painful lessons in my life. I
kept practicing, and I started reevaluating everything. All my
angers and resentments came up. I think it was all stuck in my
body. I buried all of my emotions and I didn't know that I was
doing it. I started seeing things clearly. I remembered being
seven and that my leg hurt back then. I realized that that's
where I started holding everything. With the opening of my
body, all this stuff started flowing out. I faced things head-on,
felt them, and let go. It changed me completely.

Jene R., yoga teacher

The final aim in life is *moksa,* liberation.

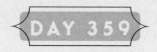

> In absorption, or *samadhi,* the witness or meditator is fully
> absorbed into the moment. There is an ecstatic experience of
> what I call the living moment. Our perspective is an unfolding,
> flowing continuum that is happening all by itself.
>
> Sudhir Jonathan Foust

As our practice deepens and expands to encompass our entire lives, we find that we are accomplishing more and more, and doing less and less. We learn to allow the same force that keeps our heart beating, digests our food for us, and maintains our health to guide us through our lives. As this process unfolds, our faith in it deepens. The love that brings peace becomes a living presence in our lives. Where once we thought and controlled, we now allow our minds to become spacious; we turn the results of our actions over to a loving universe. Our lives become an exploration in surrender. There is a new serenity in our hearts, and it shines through our eyes. We have come home, we are free.

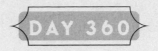

As you comb through your body for tension you learn how
to go beneath the surface of what you see, to connect
to what you feel, to the emotions inside the sensation.
When you can discern what is behind what you feel,
you can practice becoming still there.

Roman S., yoga teacher

The state of being my friend Roman is describing takes time. Most of us spend years pushing our way through our practice, managing and striving, exhilarated and disappointed, ambitious and lazy. We stay busy. We make an effort. Eventually, though, we start to take tentative steps toward getting less busy. As our attention turns inward, we discover another layer of activity. Beneath the physical sensations of our postures we discover our emotional responses. We connect at the level of *samskara,* or personality. Our habitual responses to situations become plainly visible in the stillness of our inwardly turned attention, the stillness of *samyama*. As we become still here, real change begins to happen because we are removing whatever creates the impression that we are separate. We are dissolving the false persona that obscures our true nature. We are stepping out into the light. All that is required to do this is willingness and practice. In time the clamorings of our false self grow faint and the quiet of our soul fills our lives.

S A M A D H I

DAY 361

Very often, understanding and practice do not go together.
One student may be better able to understand, while another
may have better skill in practice. In each case, he has to develop
uniformity in skill and intelligence and use them harmoniously.

B. K. S. Iyengar

B. K. S. Iyengar gives us two practical examples of imbalance. On the one hand, we can be all about action; on the other hand, we can be all about insight. At work I display elements of both. As a teacher, I am an action guy. I learn about teaching by teaching, lots of teaching. As a studio administrator, I am a visionary, an ideas man. For balance, I've learned, it is best for me to take classes from other teachers, particularly teachers with different styles. There is nothing wrong with my approach to teaching, but it always helps to get new ideas, to see other approaches. On the administration front, I know that I simply have no aptitude for implementation, so I work with a studio manager who is a details person. In no case do I take my own inclinations personally. I must be willing to see my strengths and my weaknesses, and be willing to work toward balance. Just as in asana or meditation, I must move through the stages of *samyama*. Refraining from action, I observe my reaction at the level of *samskara,* the level of personality. And then I drop down to the love that brings peace, to the place where I am open and spacious, where I invite the circumstances that will promote my spiritual health.

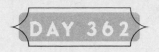
S A M A D H I

> The universe operates through dynamic exchange . . . giving
> and receiving are different aspects of the flow of energy in the
> universe. And in our willingness to give that which we seek, we
> keep the abundance of the universe circulating in our lives.
>
> Deepak Chopra

In *samyama* we become aware of life as thought and energy. The most complex physical movement is, at the same time, an idea; the most profound insight, an energetic opening. In the stillness of *samyama* we connect to the eternal dance of energy and matter—no beginning, no end. In *The Seven Spiritual Laws of Success,* Deepak Chopra stands linear thought on its head, stating that giving is receiving, and receiving is giving—no beginning, no end. This understanding has transformed my relationship to both giving and receiving. Prior to this awareness I felt guilty about receiving, and therefore experienced reluctance when giving. Because I lacked insight, my relationship to giving and receiving was tainted. I avoided both. I was blocked energetically. As a result, the world received only a small portion of what I had to offer. As my understanding shifted and my guilt fell away, I was opened up energetically. My gifts have poured out into the world, and the world's gifts have poured into my life. Time spent in *samyama* explains all of this. We connect to the real, the place where all things connect, where there is no time, no you, no me, no beginning, no end.

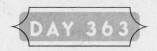

Why should a man consider himself separate? How was he
before being born or how will he be after his death? Why waste
time in such discussions? What was your form in deep sleep?
Why do you consider yourself an individual?

Talks with Ramana Maharshi

I am leaving Cambridge, Massachusetts, after eleven years. I've lived virtually all of my adult life here, most of it within the same three or four square
miles. Each street within this area has layer upon layer of memory for me.
While living here I endured the loss of my sister and fell in love with my
wife. It has been the home of my rebirth and I've never imagined leaving.
And so, as I walk down streets that are home to me, I ponder impermanence.

   We are permanence encompassed by impermanence. That part of me
which looked on in first grade looks on now. But outwardly, nothing else is
the same. My father, who only a short while ago was doing acrobatic dives
into the pool of my childhood, can no longer drive and has become quite
sick. At the level of *samskara,* of personality, I experience such change with
great wonder and sadness. I feel myself to be an individual who is losing his
home and who will lose his father someday. Louisa May Alcott wrote,
"Love is the only thing we can carry with us when we go, and it makes the
end so easy." When I step back and look at my current situation with a different perspective, I find that I am refreshed and ready, supported not by my
memories but my connection to the present. Not by a sense of how I can
protect myself from the pains of life but by a sense of how I can participate.

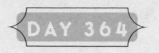
S A M A D H I

Consider [the forest lake's] silent economy and tidiness;
how the sun comes with his evaporation to sweep the
dust from its surface each morning, and a fresh
surface is constantly welling up.

Henry David Thoreau

When I drank, I would get to the end of something and I would be exhausted. There would be a tremendous push to the finish line, and then I would want to escape, to get as far away as I possibly could. I did not go to my college graduation and have been back to my alma mater only once since. I got used to things ending this way, and so it was with great surprise that at the end of my first year without a drink, I felt invigorated and eager for more. I had never experienced a completion or an ending like that. The next year, the same was true. Over time, other things started to end this way. What was once completely impossible for me has became the norm. Sober, I've been able to tap into an entirely different source of energy. Now I find that I am nourished not by the thought of something being finished, but rather by the process itself. Caught up in life, I've discovered that endings, done properly, are excellent beginnings. Having tapped into the love that brings peace, I have become like Thoreau's lake, my soul swept clean each day, a fresh surface constantly welling up.

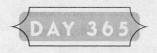

> From mastery of *samyama* comes the light
> of awareness and insight.
>
> Yoga Sutras

The four aims of life are not fulfilled by yoga; they are fulfilled by our actions, by the choices that we make each day. The intention of yoga is to give us a place to start, and sustenance for our journey. Nothing is wasted. Every ability we foster in our practice of yoga supports the living of a full life. The clarity, insight, and equanimity we derive from the consistent experience of *samyama* provides the basis upon which both wisdom and creativity can flourish in our lives. Effectiveness, health, and lightness of heart are the concrete results of our practice.

I have had the good fortune of witnessing the truth of this in the lives of thousands of people over a number of years. I have watched as people have endured sickness and loss, good times and bad. In my own life, too, there have been many cycles of death and rebirth. Through it all, yoga has been the still point for me and for those around me. Yoga is the place to which we always return, to connect to what's real and to let love weave its way through the fabric of our lives. The only mistake I have ever seen a person make on this path is to stop practicing.

At the beginning of this book I invited you to get into the canoe of your practice and ride down the river of life. I hope you are still paddling as you read these words and that we will meet some sunny day out on the river of life. Until then . . . *Namaste!*

PART EIGHT

·Self-Forgetting

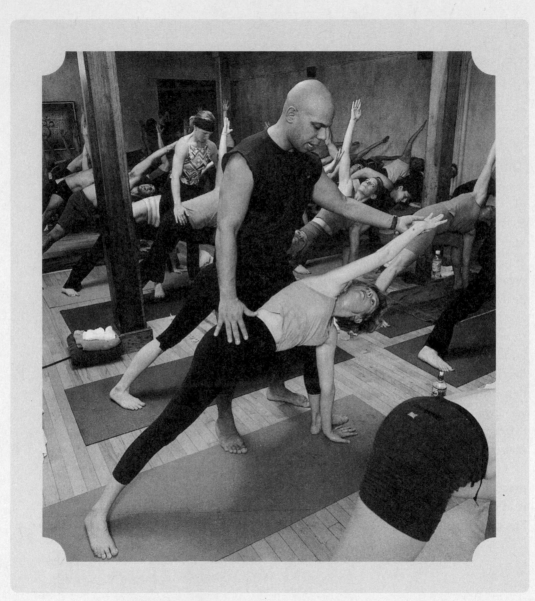

We show up, burn brightly in the moment,
live passionately, and when the moment is over,
when our work is done, we step back and let go.

Victory to our spirits, peace to all beings.

REFERENCE LIST

Alcoholics Anonymous. New York: Alcoholics Anonymous World Services, Inc., 1939, 1955, 1976.

Allen, David. *Getting Things Done: The Art of Stress-Free Productivity.* New York: Viking, 2001.

Anderson, Peggy, comp. *Great Quotes from Great Leaders.* New Jersey: The Career Press Inc., 1997.

As Bill Sees It. New York: Alcoholics Anonymous World Services, Inc., 1967.

Barks, Coleman, and Michael Green. *The Illuminated Prayer: The Five-Times Prayer of the Sufis as Revealed by Jellaludin Rumi and Bawa Muhaiyaddeen.* New York: A Ballantine Wellspring Book, The Ballantine Publishing Group, 2000.

Barks, Coleman, with John Moyne, trans. *The Essential Rumi.* Edison, New Jersey: Castle Books, 1995, 1997.

Birch, Beryl Bender. *Beyond Power Yoga.* New York: A Fireside Book, Simon & Schuster, 2000.

Birch, Beryl Bender. *Power Yoga.* New York: A Fireside Book, Simon & Schuster, 1995.

Bradshaw, John. *Healing the Shame that Binds You.* Deerfield Beach, Florida: Health Communications, Inc., 1988.

Cameron, Julia. *Heart Steps: Prayers and Declarations for a Creative Life.* New York: Jeremy P. Tarcher/Putnam, 1997.

Carter-Scott, Cherie. *If Success Is a Game, These Are the Rules.* New York: Bantam Doubleday Dell Publishing, 2000.

Chodron, Pema. *The Places that Scare You: A Guide to Fearlessness in Difficult Times.* Boston: Shambhala Publications, 1994.

Chodron, Pema. *Start Where You Are: A Guide to Compassionate Living.* Boston: Shambhala Publications, 2001.

Chodron, Pema. *When Things Fall Apart: Heart Advice for Difficult Times.* Boston: Shambhala Publications, 1997.

Chodron, Pema. *The Wisdom of No Escape: And the Path of Loving-kindness.* Boston: Shambhala Publications, 1991.

Chopra, Deepak. *How to Know God: The Soul's Journey into the Mystery of Mysteries.* New York: Three Rivers Press, 2000.

Chopra, Deepak. *The Path to Love: Renewing the Power of Spirit in Your Life.* New York: Harmony Books, 1997.

Chopra, Deepak. *The Seven Spiritual Laws of Success: A Practical Guide to the Fulfillment of Your Dreams.* New York: Amber-Allen Publishing, 1995.

Coelho, Paul. *The Fifth Mountain.* New York: HarperCollins Publishers, 1998.

Coelho, Paul. *The Pilgrimage.* London: HarperCollins Publishers, 1987.

Cohen, M. J. *The Penguin Thesaurus of Quotations.* England: Penguin Books, 1998.

Cope, Stephen. *Yoga and the Quest for the True Self.* New York: Bantam Books, 1999.

A Course in Miracles. Tiburon, California: Foundation for Inner Peace, 1975.

A Course in Miracles Workbook for Students. Tiburon, California: Foundation for Inner Peace, 1975.

Covey, Stephen R. *The 7 Habits of Highly Effective People: Powerful Lessons in Personal Change.* New York: A Fireside Book, Simon and Schuster, 1989.

Das, Ram, and Mirabai Bush. *Compassion in Action, Setting out on the Path of Service.* New York: Bell Tower, 1992.

Das, Surya Lama. *Awakening the Buddha Within: Tibetan Wisdom for the Western World.* New York: Broadway Books, 1997.

De Mello, Anthony. *The Way to Love: The Last Meditations of Anthony De Mello.* New York: An Image Book, Doubleday, 1991.

Farhi, Donna. *The Breathing Book.* New York: An Owl Book, Henry Holt and Company LLC, 1996.

Farhi, Donna. *Yoga Mind, Body & Spirit: A Return to Wholeness.* New York: An Owl Book, Henry Holt and Company LLC, 2000.

Feuerstein, Georg, Ph.D. *The Yoga Tradition: Its History, Literature, Philosophy and Practice.* Prescott, Arizona: Hohm Press, 1998.

Feuerstein, Georg, Ph.D., and Stephan Bodian with the staff of *Yoga Journal. Living Yoga: A Comprehensive Guide for Daily Life.* New York: Jeremy P. Tarcher/ Putnam, 1993.

Feuerstein, Georg, Ph.D., and Jeanine Miller. *The Essence of Yoga*. Rochester, Vermont: Inner Traditions International, 1971, 1998.

Fields, Rick, Peggy Taylor, Rex Weyler, and Rick Ingrasci. *Chop Wood Carry Water*. New York: Jeremy P. Tarcher/Putnam Books, 1984.

Gladwell, Malcolm. *The Tipping Point: How Little Things Can Make a Big Difference*. Boston/New York/London: Little, Brown and Company, 2000.

Gibran, Kahlil. *The Prophet*. New York: Alfred A. Knopf, Inc., 1923.

Gibran, Kahlil. *Sand & Foam*. New York: Alfred A. Knopf, Inc., 1926.

Hanh, Thich Nhat. *The Heart of Understanding*. Edited by Peter Levitt. Berkeley, California: Parallax Press, 1988.

Hanh, Thich Nhat. *The Miracle of Mindfulness*. Translated by Mobi Ho. Boston: Beacon Press, 1975.

Harvey, Andrew. *Son to Man: The Mystical Path to Christ*. New York: Jeremy P. Tarcher/Putnam, 1998.

Hesse, Hermann. *Siddhartha*. New York: New Directions Publishing Corporation, 1951.

Hoff, Benjamin. *The Tao of Pooh*. London & New York: Penguin Books, 1982.

Holleman, Dona, and Orit Sen-Gupta. *Dancing the Body of Light*. New York: Pandion Enterprise, 1999.

The Holy Bible—Revised Standard Edition. Philadelphia & New York: A. J. Holman Company, (Old Testament Section: Copyright 1952. New Testament Section, First Edition: Copyright 1946. New Testament Section, Second Edition: Copyright 1971).

Hugo, Victor. *Les Miserables*. New York: Modern Library, 1992.

Iyengar, B. K. S. *Light on Yoga*. New York: Schocken Books, 1966.

Iyengar, B. K. S. *Light on the Yoga Sutras of Patanjali*. London: Thorsons, 1993.

Iyengar, B. K. S. *The Tree of Yoga*. Boston: Shambhala Publications, Inc., 1988.

Johnson, Spencer, M.D. *Who Moved My Cheese?* New York: G. P. Putnam's Sons, 1998.

Johnston, Charles, trans., (and commentary). *Yoga Sutras of Patanjali*. Albuquerque, New Mexico, 1912.

Jois, Sri K. Pattabhi. *Yoga Mala*. New York: Eddie Stern/Patanjali Yoga Shala, 1999.

Juhan, Deane. *Job's Body: A Handbook for Bodywork*. Barrytown, New York: Barrytown Ltd., 1998.

Kennedy, John F. *Profiles in Courage*. New York: Harper & Brothers, 1956.

King, Dr. Martin Luther, Jr. *Where Do We Go from Here: Chaos or Community?* Boston: Beacon Press, 1967.

King, Stephen. *On Writing*. New York: Pocket Books, 2000.

Kornfield, Jack. *After the Ecstasy, the Laundry*. New York: Bantam Books, 2000.

Krishnamurti, J. *Think on These Things*. New York: Harper Perennial, 1989.

Lasater, Judith, Ph.D., P.T. *Living Your Yoga: Finding the Spiritual in Everyday Life*. Berkeley, California: Rodmell Press, 2000.

Maitreya, Balangoda Ananda (The Venerable), trans. *The Dhammapada: The Path of Truth*. Berkley: Parallax Press, 1995. (Originally published by Lotsawa Publications, 1988).

Masters, Roy, and Mel Tappan. *How to Conquer Negative Emotions*. California: Foundation of Human Understanding, 1975.

Merzel, Dennis Genpo. *24/7 Dharma*. Boston/Tokyo/Singapore: Journey Editions, 2001.

Miller, Richard, C. Ph.D. *Breathing for Life: Articles on the Art and Science of the Breath*. (Series of articles.) Sebastopol, California: Anahata Press.

Millman, Dan. *Way of the Peaceful Warrior*. Tiburon, California: H. J. Kramer, Inc., 1980.

Mitchell, Stephen. *Bhagavad Gita: A New Translation*. New York: Harmony Books, 2000.

Mitchell, Stephen. *Tao Te Ching: A New English Version*. New York: Harper Perennial, 1992.

Mother Teresa. *No Greater Love*. Edited by Becky Benenate and Joseph Durepos. Novato, California: New World Library, 1997.

Myers, Tom. *Anatomy Trains*. Edinburgh: Churchill Livingston, 2001.

Oliver, Mary. *The Leaf and the Cloud: A Poem*. Cambridge: Da Capo Press, 2001.

Peterson, Jesse Lee. *From Rage to Responsibility*. St. Paul, Minnesota: Paragon House, 2000.

Reps, Paul, and Nyogen Senzaki, comps. *Zen Flesh Zen Bones.* Boston, Rutland, VT/ Tokyo: Tuttle Publishing, 1957. (1957, 1985 Charles E. Tuttle Company, Inc.)

Rinpoche, Sogyal. *The Tibetan Book of Living and Dying.* San Francisco: HarperSan-Francisco, 1993.

Ruiz, Don Miguel. *The Four Agreements: A Practical Guide to Personal Freedom, A Toletic Wisdom Book.* New York: Amber-Allen Publishing, 2001.

Safransky, Sy, ed. *Sunbeams: A Book of Quotations.* Berkeley, California: North Atlantic Books, 1990.

Schiffmann, Erich. *Yoga: The Spirit and Practice of Moving into Stillness.* New York: Pocket Books, 1996.

Sinh, Pancham, trans. *The Hatha Yoga Pradipika.* New Delhi, India: Oriental Books Reprint Corporation, 1914. (First published by Panini Office, Allahabad, 1914).

Steinem, Gloria. *Moving Beyond Words.* New York: Simon & Schuster, 1994.

Talks with Ramana Maharshi: On Realizing Abiding Peace and Happiness. Carlsbad, California: Inner Directions Foundation, 2000. (All of the talks were recorded by Sri Munagala S. Venkataramiah (Swami Ramanananda) but he is not listed as editor. Foreword is by Ken Wilbur.)

Tanakh: A New Translation of the Holy Scriptures. Philadelphia/Jerusalem: The Jewish Publication Society, 1993.

Thoreau, Henry David. *Walking.* New York: HarperSanFrancisco, 1994.

Thurman, Howard. *Jesus and the Disinherited.* Boston: Beacon Press, 1976.

Thurman, Robert. *Inner Revolution: Life, Liberty and the Pursuit of Real Happiness.* New York: Riverhead Books, 1998.

Tolle, Eckhart. *The Power of Now: A Guide to Spiritual Enlightenment.* Novato, California: New World Library, 1999.

The Twelve Steps and Twelve Traditions of Alcoholics Anonymous. New York: Alcoholics Anonymous World Services, Inc., 1952.

Vivekananda, Swami. *Raja-Yoga.* New York: Ramakrishna Vivekananda Center, 1956.

Williamson, Angel Kyodo. *Being Black: Zen and the Art of Living with Fearlessness and Grace.* New York: Viking Compass, 2000.

Williamson, Marianne. *A Return to Love: Reflections on the Principles of A Course in Miracles.* New York: HarperCollins Publishers, 1992.

Yogananda, Paramahansa. *Autobiography of a Yogi.* Los Angeles, California: Self-Realization Fellowship, 1946 (Copyright renewed by SRF in 1974, 1981 & 1994).

Zaleski, Philip, ed. *The Best Spiritual Writing 2000.* New York: HarperSanFrancisco, 2000.

ABOUT THE AUTHORS

Born in Manhattan, ROLF GATES grew up in the Boston area and attended American University in Washington, D.C. In 1987 he received a degree in American history and his commission in the U.S. Army Infantry from Georgetown University. As a military officer he became an Airborne Ranger and served with U.S. forces in Germany. Since then he has worked as an emergency medical technician and an addictions counselor, specializing in adolescents in residential programs. In 1997 he became certified to teach Kripalu yoga. Gates directed the Baptiste Power Yoga Studio in Cambridge for three years and now co-owns and directs Baptiste Power Yoga, The Boston Studio, in Boston, MA. In addition to his weekly teaching schedule he is responsible for the supervision and professional development of the teaching staff of the Boston and Cambridge studios. He appears regularly modeling yoga poses in *Natural Health* magazine and has conducted workshops throughout the United States and abroad. In 2002, he was named "Best Yoga Teacher" by *Boston Magazine.* He lives in Boston with his wife, yoga teacher Mariam Gates.

KATRINA KENISON has been the annual editor of *The Best American Short Stories* since 1990. In 1999 she was coeditor, with John Updike, of the national best-seller *The Best American Short Stories of the Century.* She co-edited the anthology *Mothers: Twenty Stories of Contemporary Motherhood* and is the author of *Mitten Strings for God: Reflections for Mothers in a Hurry.* Her essays and articles have appeared in *O, The Oprah Magazine,* where she has been a contributing editor, and in *Redbook, Ladies' Home Journal, Family Circle,* and *Family Life.* Kenison lives outside Boston with her husband, Steven Lewers, and their two sons. She began practicing yoga with Rolf Gates in 2000.